Clinical Research in Gastroenterology 2

Clinical Research in Gastroenterology 2

edited by

S. Matern
Director of the Third Department of Internal Medicine
Medical Faculty of Aachen University of Technology
Aachen, FRG

KLUWER ACADEMIC PUBLISHERS
DORDRECHT / BOSTON / LONDON

Distributors

---

for the United States and Canada: Kluwer Academic Publishers, PO Box 358, Accord Station, Hingham, MA 02018-0358, USA
for all other countries: Kluwer Academic Publishers Group, Distribution Center, PO Box 322, 3300 AH Dordrecht, The Netherlands

British Library Cataloguing in Publication Data

Clinical research in gastroenterology.
2.
1. Man. Gastrointestinal tract. Diseases
I. Matern, S. (Siegfried)
616.3'3

ISBN-13: 978-94-010-7622-7 e-ISBN-13: 978-94-009-2488-8
DOI: 10.1007/978-94-009-2488-8

Published in the United Kingdom by Kluwer Academic Publishers, PO Box 55, Lancaster, UK.

Kluwer Academic Publishers BV incorporates the publishing programmes of D. Reidel, Martinus Nijhoff, Dr W. Junk and MTP Press.

Contents

List of Contributors

R. Bares
Department of Nuclear Medicine
Technical University of Aachen
Aachen, FRG

M. Betzler
Department of Surgery
University of Heidelberg
Heidelberg, FRG

R. Büchsel
Department of Internal Medicine III
Technical University of Aachen
Pauwelstrasse
5100 Aachen, FRG

U. Buell
Department of Nuclear Medicine
Technical University of Aachen
Aachen, FRG

A. Gangl
1. Department of Gastroenterology
and Hepatology
University of Vienna
Lazarettgasse 14, A-1090 Vienna
Austria

C. Herfarth
Department of Surgery
University of Heidelberg
Heidelberg, FRG

U. Klotz
Dr Margarete Fischer-Bosch-
Institute of Clinical Pharmacology
Stuttgart, FRG

H. Lochs
1. Department of Gastroenterology
and Hepatology
University of Vienna
Lazarettgasse 14, A-1090 Vienna
Austria

S. Matern
Department of Internal Medicine III
Technical University of Aachen
Pauwelstrasse
5100 Aachen, FRG

J. Schölmerich
Department of Internal Medicine
University of Freiburg
Hugstetter Str. 55
7800 Freiburg, FRG

H.J. Thon
Department of Internal Medicine III
Technical University of Aachen
Pauwelstrasse
5100 Aachen, FRG

H. Wietholtz
Department of Internal Medicine III
Technical University of Aachen
Pauwelstrasse
5100 Aachen, FRG

Preface

Inflammatory bowel disease – i.e. ulcerative colitis and Crohn's disease – not only creates significant patient morbidity but also imposes a diagnostic and therapeutic challenge to the physician in charge of these patients.

Since the development of sulphasalazine by Dr Nanna Svartz in Sweden half a century ago, important improvements in the prognosis of ulcerative colitis and Crohn's disease have been achieved. This book makes an attempt to present and discuss some of the most recent advances in diagnostic procedures and therapeutic approaches to inflammatory bowel disease with special respect to Crohn's disease.

Although the final diagnosis of ulcerative colitis and Crohn's disease is generally based on endoscopic, histological or X-ray examinations, nuclear medicine and its imaging procedures have established their place in certain aspects of inflammatory bowel disease. One chapter of this book is dedicated accordingly to the indications of nuclear diagnostic procedures in the clinical setting.

Sulphasalazine has been the mainstay of medical therapy in ulcerative colitis and Crohn's disease of the colon. Recently 5-aminosalicylic acid has been discovered to be its active compound and sulphapyridine was found to be the component responsible for most of the adverse effects of sulphasalazine. It is not surprising that many studies have investigated 5-aminosalicylic acid as a single therapeutic agent in inflammatory bowel disease. Several new preparations of 5-aminosalicylic acid offer great potential in the treatment of ulcerative colitis and Crohn's disease. For this reason the clinical pharmacology of 5-aminosalicylic acid in inflammatory bowel disease and the possibilities of medical therapy in Crohn's disease is presented here.

Malnutrition and disturbance of intestinal absorption are major problems that frequently complicate inflammatory bowel disease in patients of all ages. The dietary management of inflammatory bowel disease has elicited variable interest among clinicians over the years. At present there is increasing evidence for a significant role of nutritional therapy in the management of patients with Crohn's disease. Therefore the role of nutritional therapy as well as the effect of supplementary therapy on extraintestinal symptoms of Crohn's disease is discussed.

Most patients with Crohn's disease will require one or more operations during the course of their disease. Surgery of Crohn's disease is not curative but offers elective palliation for a variety of complications. The growing tendency for early operation prompted the chapter on the current state of surgery in Crohn's disease.

I want to thank those who have participated in this volume for their contributions on their individual fields of expertise. Finally I want to acknowledge gratefully the assistance of Mr Phil Johnstone and Dr Peter Clarke from Kluwer Academic Publishers who made this book possible with great patience and excellent organization.

Siegfried Matern

1
Nuclear medicine procedures in diagnosing inflammatory bowel disease

R. BARES AND U. BUELL

INTRODUCTION

Diagnostic procedures in inflammatory bowel disease should provide information about:

Type of disease (Crohn's disease, ulcerative colitis, etc.)
Localization
Activity grading
Complications (abscesses, fistulae, joint disease)
Disorders of bowel function.

The final diagnosis is usually made by endoscopy (gastroduodenoscopy, colonoscopy) including histology of biopsied specimen or by X-ray examinations (barium meal and enema, enteroclysis, abdominal computed tomography). In addition, an increasing number of nuclear procedures is available which, in contrast to morphologically focussed endoscopic and radiographic methods, aim to reveal functional data. The goal of this review is to introduce these nuclear methods and then to figure out indications for their employment in the clinical routine.

In general nuclear diagnostic methods may be subdivided into imaging and non-imaging procedures. In diagnosing inflammatory bowel disease, one group of imaging procedures is used to localize the inflammation, a second to evaluate the functional sequelae (Table 1.1).

Table 1.1 Nuclear diagnostic methods in inflammatory bowel disease

Imaging procedures
Localization of inflammatory bowel disease
Leukocyte scanning
^{67}Ga scintigraphy
Other methods
Evaluation of functional disorders and extraintestinal disease
Intestinal transit studies
Bone scintigraphy
Non-imaging procedures
Intestinal absorption of bile acids
Absorption of ^{75}Se-homotaurocholic acid (SeHCAT)
Absorption of ^{14}C-taurocholic acid (TCA)
Absorption of ^{14}C-glycocholic acid and breath test
Intestinal absorption of vitamin B_{12}
Intestinal permeability
Intestinal protein exudation

IMAGING PROCEDURES

Localization of inflammatory bowel disease

Leukocyte scanning

In vitro labelling of human leukocytes with ^{111}In-oxine was introduced into clinical practice in 1976 by Thakur and McAffee[1–4]. Briefly, they performed several centrifugations to obtain leukocyte-rich plasma which was finally incubated with 8–17 MBq ^{111}In-oxine. Reported labelling efficiency is 50–80%.

After labelling the leukocyte preparation has to be reinjected intravenously. Scintigrams of the abdominal and pelvic area are usually acquired 4 and 24 h later. In healthy patients no radioactivity can be seen within the intestine. In the case of active inflammatory bowel disease, early images 4 h post injection reveal foci of leukocyte accumulation suggestive of inflammation. At these locations labelled leukocytes are excreted into the bowel and transported distally by peristalsis which can be demonstrated on delayed images 24 h post injection. The extent of leukocyte excretion reflects the disease activity. Quantitative assessment is possible by measuring 24-h faecal collections in a gamma counter (recovery of more than 2% of the injected radioactivity proves active disease[5,6]).

In intra-abdominal abscesses, the accumulation of radiolabelled leukocytes does not change place between 4 and 24 h post injection. No radioactivity is found within the bowel unless additional inflammatory bowel disease exists[7,8].

Recently modified labelling techniques have been described for achieving preparations of pure granulocytes[9,10] or using lipophilic ^{99m}Tc-hexamethylpropyleneamine oxime (HMPAO) for leukocyte labelling[11]. As with ^{111}In-oxine, however, time-consuming (about 2 h) separation procedures which require skilled personnel and sophisticated instrumentation have to be accommodated. In the future these may be replaced by the application of radiolabelled monoclonal antibodies directed against granulocyte antigens[12,13].

Gallium-67 scintigraphy

Intravenously administered ^{67}Ga-citrate accumulates in abscesses and low-grade inflammations[14]. Although this compound is easy to handle and has been well known for about 20 years it has become less important since leukocyte scanning was introduced. The reasons for this are later examination periods (48–72 h), an unspecific mechanism of accumulation, and the fairly high radiation exposure of the patients.

Other methods

In 1979 Kadir[15] reported uptake of intravenously administered ^{99m}Tc DTPA in inflammatory bowel lesions. Recently this was confirmed by Abdel-Dayem and coworkers[16] in a small number of patients. More data, especially concerning the mechanism of accumulation, are necessary to evaluate this new technique.

Sucralphate is a well-known drug for treatment of peptic ulcerations. After *in vitro* labelling with ^{99m}Tc[17,18], it can be used for detection of mucosal damages within the intestine. Following oral application, the labelled compound passes through the gastrointestinal tract by peristalsis and may adhere to mucosal lesions if present. Clinical studies in patients with oesophagitis, gastric and duodenal ulcerations, yielded positive results;

findings in patients with inflammatory bowel disease, however, have so far been controversial[19,20].

Evaluation of functional disorders and extraintestinal disease

Intestinal transit studies

Intestinal transit can be measured following oral administration of radio-labelled test meals. The markers used (^{99m}Tc-DTPA or ^{111}In-DTPA for liquids, ^{99m}Tc sulphur colloid for solid food – labelled eggs, chicken liver, etc.) should be stable, non-adhesive to intestinal mucosa and not be absorbed during their passage[21]. The calculated transit times between different parts of the intestine characterize the transport of food and its fragments[22] and provide quantitative data about motility disorders. Alterations in gastric emptying, especially, can be assessed accurately and correlated with malnourishment in patients with inflammatory bowel disease[23].

Bone scintigraphy

Inflammatory bowel disease is accompanied by extraintestinal manifestations in about 19% of all patients, especially arthritis/arthralgia[24–26]. Therefore, bone scintigraphy with ^{99m}Tc-labelled phosphonates is a useful screening method, if patients present symptoms suggestive for joint disease. Positive findings are characterized by elevated tracer uptake in the suspected joint. Quantitative data exist for the sacroiliac joints in particular[27].

NON-IMAGING PROCEDURES

Intestinal absorption of bile acids

Absorption of ^{75}selenium-homotaurocholic acid

^{75}Selenium-homotaurocholic acid (SeHCAT), a synthetic conjugated bile acid, is labelled in the 24-C position with ^{75}Se. After oral administration it is quantitatively absorbed by active, ionic transport while passing the terminal ileum[28]. The extent of passive non-ionic diffusion is unimportant. As SeHCAT is nearly completely excreted into the bile, its retention within the body depends mainly on ileal resorption, ie. on the functional integrity of the ileum. SeHCAT retention can be measured using a whole-body counter or uncollimated gamma camera[29,30]. To achieve optimal sensitivity, the test should be extended until the seventh day following application[31]. Pathological results, however, are often gained as early as 20–30 h p.c.[32]. Figure 1.1A and B show SeHCAT distribution 1 and 3 h p.c., Figure 1.2 demonstrates the time course of SeHCAT retention in a healthy control and in patients with ileal Crohn's disease or resected ileum.

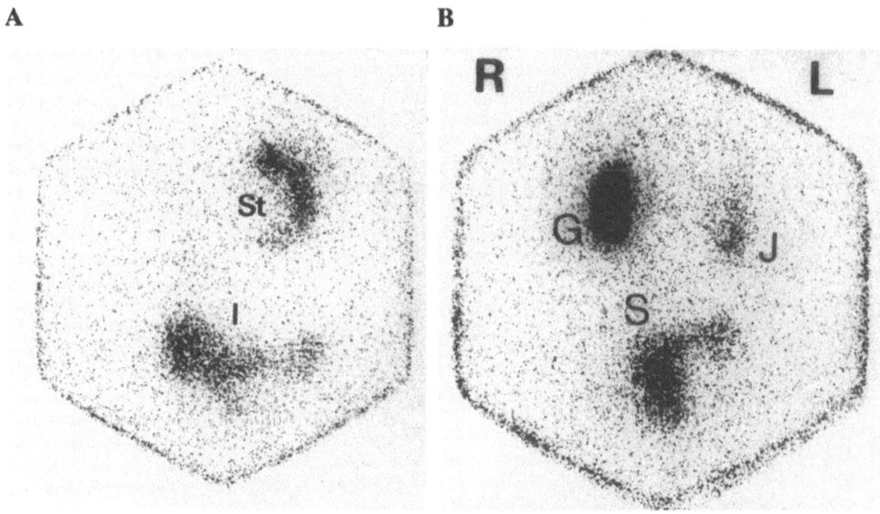

Figure 1.1 SeHCAT distribution: (A, left) 1 h following oral administration. About half of the radiolabelled bile acid has reached the ileum (I) while the second half still remains within the stomach (St); (B, right) 3 h p.c.. Note that most of the radioactivity is now located in the gallbladder (G). A smaller amount which has not been absorbed has reached the rectosigmoid area (S), and a little can be detected in the jejunum (J) having passed the enterohepatic circulation

Absorption of ^{14}C-taurocholic acid

After oral or intravenous application, taurine-conjugated cholic acid labelled with ^{14}C joins the physiologic bile acid pool. Like SeHCAT it is actively absorbed in the ileum, but is also passively absorbed in the large bowel by non-ionic diffusion. Faecal excretion of ^{14}C, measured according to the method of Lindstedt[33], yields quantitative data concerning the faecal loss of cholic acid.

Absorption of ^{14}C-glycocholic acid and breath test

Like SeHCAT and ^{14}C-TCA, cholic acid conjugated with ^{14}C-labelled glycine is absorbed by active transport in the ileum and passively in the large bowel after bacterial deconjugation. In pathological states (bacterial overgrowth of the small bowel) passive diffusion also takes place within the jejunum and ileum following deconjugation. The ^{14}C-labelled glycine will be released intraluminally and rapidly converted to $^{14}CO_2$, which in turn will be absorbed and expired[34].

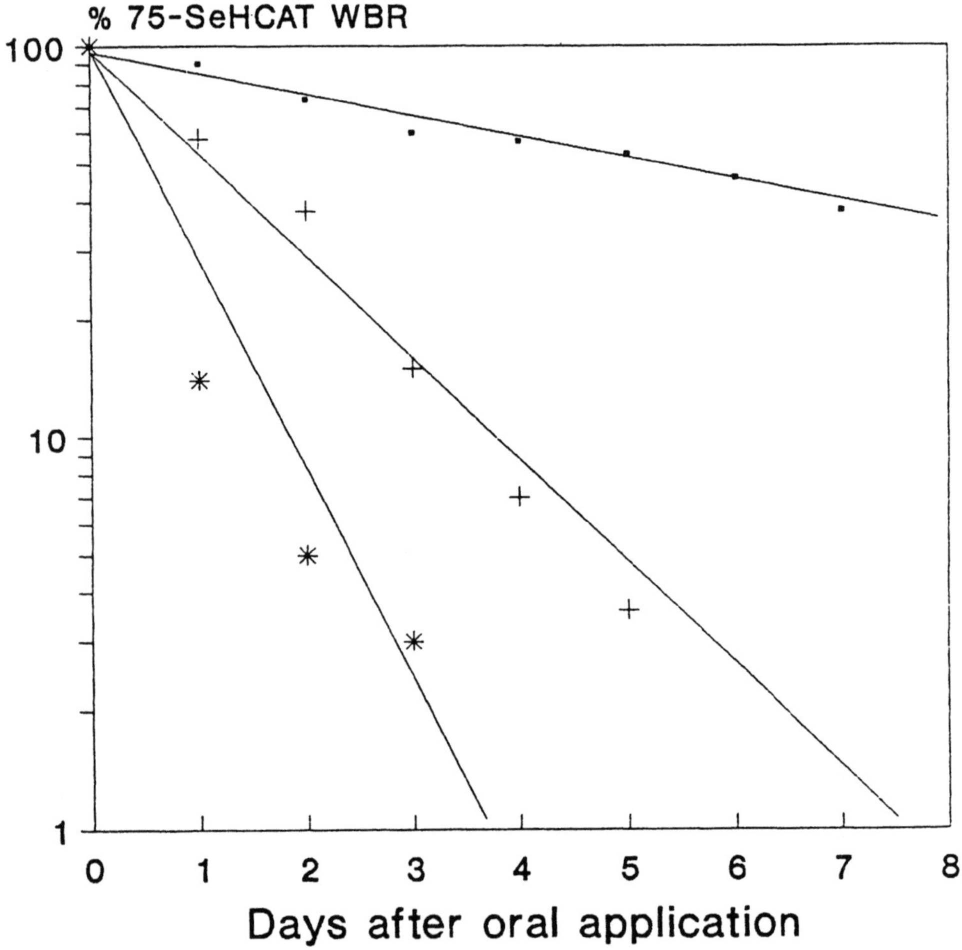

Figure 1.2 Time course of ^{75}SeHCAT retention (logarithmic scale) in three patients: • = without inflammatory bowel disease; + = suffering ileal Crohn's disease; * = after ileal resection

The absorption of ^{14}C-glycocholic acid can be assessed by measurement of the faecal excretion – similar to the method of Lindstedt[33]. The breath test, as described by Fromm and Hoffmann[35], gives quantitative information about bacterial deconjugation in small and large bowel, which can be discriminated by the time course of the $^{14}CO_2$ excretion in breath[34].

Intestinal absorption of vitamin B_{12}

Mediated by intrinsic factor (IF), vitamin B_{12} is physiologically absorbed in the terminal ileum by active transport. The functional integrity of the ileum may therefore be assessed by measuring the absorption of ^{58}Co-labelled vitamin B_{12}, if a deficit of innnnnntriiinsic factor or bacterial overgrowth (which dstroys the vitamin B_{12}–IF complex. The urinary excretion test of Schilling[32], which assesses the recovery of orally applied ^{58}Co-labelled vitamin B_{12} in a 24-h urine collection, has become an accepted method in clinical routine.

Intestinal permeability

Absorption of ^{51}Cr-labelled ethylenediamine tetraacetate (EDTA) depends on intestinal permeability and can be evaluated by measurement of urinary excretion of the orally applied compound[36,37]. In animal studies, increased excretion was found in small bowel inflammation while colonic disease yielded normal results. This might be due to its smaller surface compared with small bowel[37].

Intestinal protein exudation

Various diseases, especially inflammatory bowel diseases, cause abnormal exudation of serum proteins into the intestine. The extent of exudation can be assessed by faecal radioactivity measurements following intravenous administration of radiolabelled proteins (^{51}Cr-albumin, ^{59}Fe-dextran)[38,39].

CLINICAL RESULTS

Crohn's disease

In clinical routine the diagnosis of Crohn's disease is established by endoscopy (including biopsies) and X-ray examinations. Both provide precise morphological information about the large bowel and upper gastrointestinal tract. The evaluation of jejunum and ileum, however, is often difficult since it is based mainly on radiological findings which are of limited sensitivity and specificity[40]. In these situations nuclear methods may gain importance. Applied to patients with indecisive morphological findings, leukocyte scanning gives accurate information about localization of inflamed bowel segments[5,10,41–43]. The reported sensitivities vary between 90 and 100%. Results of comparative studies between leukocyte scanning and endoscopy are reviewed in Table 1.2. Figure 1.3 shows a typical scan obtained in ileal Crohn's disease.

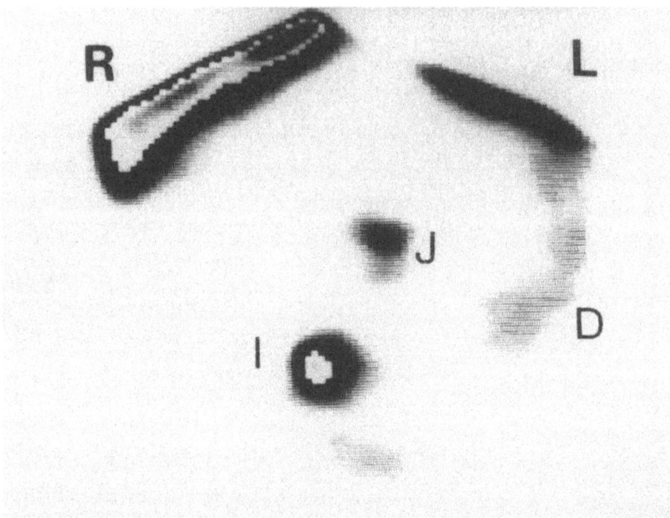

Figure 1.3 ^{111}In scan (courtesy of A. Wicke): anterior view obtained 24 h after reinjection of autologous granulocytes in a patient with confirmed Crohn's disease. Note localized granulocyte accumulation within the jejunum (J) and ileum (I) and transport of excreted granulocytes to the descending colon (D)

For clinical assessment the Crohn's disease activity index (CDAI) was developed by Best and coworkers[46,47]. Though this index has proven its usefulness it is known that symptoms often occur and change with delay[24].

Therefore, an objective and sensitive assessment of disease activity is desirable. This can be achieved with a sensitivity of 97% and a specificity of 100% by measuring faecal excretion of ^{111}In-labelled leukocytes[48]. As a simple alternative, measurements of SeHCAT retention allow a quantitative evaluation of the absorptive function of the terminal ileum. Merrick[31] detected compromised SeHCAT resorption in ileal Crohn's disease with a

Table 1.2 Results of ^{111}In leukocyte scanning compared with endoscopical and radiological findings in Crohn's disease

Author	*No. of patients*	*No. of lesions*	*Sensitivity (%)*	*Specificity (%)*
Becker[5]	31 [a]	27 [b]	90	85
Saverymuttu[42]	37	37 [b]	100	100
Saverymuttu[43]	24	24 [b]	94	100
Stein[44]	5	25	92	77
Ybern[45]	11	18	94	100

[a] Includes patients with Crohn's disease, ulcerative colitis, *Yersinia* enteritis, and Whipple's disease.
[b] Exact number of lesions not specified.

sensitivity of 78% and specificity of 86%. False-negative results may occur if stenotic ileal segments cause a delayed SeHCAT transit through the intestine[49]. A summary of the results of faecal leukocyte excretion and SeHCAT retention measurements compared with surgical, endoscopical and radiological findings is given in Tables 1.3 and 1.4.

A further diagnostic problem is the detection of abscesses and fistulae. The latter may be confirmed by use of contrast media in X-ray examinations. Localization of intra-abdominal abscesses, however, is difficult, even if ultrasonography and/or computerized tomography are employed (sensitivity 60–82% and 86–95%, respectively[8,51,53,54]. In such cases leukocyte scanning is able to localize and differentiate abscesses from inflammations with a sensitivity of about 95% and specificity of about 99%[7,8,55].

Functional changes caused by Crohn's disease are hardly recognized by endoscopy or X-ray examinations. Reduced ileal resorption, altered permeability of the bowel wall, and bacterial overgrowth, are exclusively measured by nuclear procedures (SeHCAT absorption, renal excretion of ^{51}Cr-EDTA, ^{14}C-glycocholic acid breath test). Thus, they may provide important data for selecting an adequate therapy in malabsorptive syndromes, bile acid loss and chologenic diarrhoea[31,35,36,47,56].

Table 1.3 Faecal excretion of ^{111}In-labelled leukocytes compared with endoscopical and radiological findings in patients with Crohn's disease

Author	*No. of patients*	*Sensitivity (%)*	*Specificity (%)*
Becker[5]	31	100	100
Saverymuttu[42]	37	100	100[a]
Saverymuttu[43]	24	97	100

[a] Agreement with clinical evaluation in 10/12 patients.

Table 1.4 Results of SeHCAT retention compared with endoscopical/radiological findings and vitamin B_{12} absorption in patients with Crohn's disease

Author	*No. of patients*	*Normal limit*	*Compromised retention in:* *ICD*	*Res*	*CCD*	*UC*	*Ctr*	*Compromised absorption of vitamin B_{12}*
Fagan[50]	30	>6% D7	6/6	8/8	0/3	0/3	0/10	14/14
Holdstock[30]	44	>19% D7	9/14	9/9	2/10	0/11	0	
Merrick[31]	279	>19% D7	sensitivity 78%		specificity 86%		accuracy 90%	
Nyhlin[51]	62	>12% D7	6/6	8/8		2/16	0/17	6/11
Scheurlen[49]	31	T50%>28h	5/5	5/5	0/8	0/8	1/5	
Thaysen[52]	28	>30% D7	6/6			0/4	7/28	
Bares[b]	25	>19% D7	4/7[a]	6/6	0/3	1/2	5/7	3/12

Abbreviations: ICD = ileal Crohn's disease, Res = ileal resection, CCD = colonic Crohn's disease, UC = ulcerative colitis, Ctr = controls.
[a] Including three patients with ileal stenosis.
[b] Unpublished data.

Ulcerative colitis

Ulcerative colitis can be diagnosed accurately only by colonoscopy providing specimen for histological evaluation. Nuclear localizing procedures, especially leukocyte scanning, are useful if endoscopy cannot be performed (critically ill patients) or barium enema reveals indecisive findings. The reported sensitivity of leukocyte scanning in ulcerative colitis is close to 100%[10,48]. A specific diagnosis, however, as differentiation of ulcerative colitis *vs* Crohn's disease *vs* colorectal carcinoma, cannot be obtained. Table 1.5 reviews results of leukocyte scanning compared to endoscopical and radiological findings. As in Crohn's disease, the activity of ulcerative colitis can be assessed objectively by counting faecal radioactivity[5,6].

Ileal bile absorption is usually within normal limits. Inflammatory involvement of the ascending colon, however, is reported to lead to an increased excretion of ^{14}C-TCA[57]. As in Crohn's disease measurements of protein exudation reveal pathological results.

Table 1.5 Results of ^{111}In leukocyte scanning compared to endoscopical and radiological findings in patients with ulcerative colitis

Author	*No. of patients*	*No. of lesions*	*Sensitivity (%)*	*Specificity (%)*
Becker[5]	7	7 [a]	100	100
Saverymuttu[48]	7	7 [a]	100	100
Saverymuttu[43]	9	9 [a]	89	100
Stein[44]	10	50	80	7 false positive
Ybern[45]	16	14 [a]	79	100

[a] Exact number of lesions not specified.

Various inflammatory bowel diseases

In patients with abdominal complaints leukocyte scanning can confirm the type of disease (inflammatory, e.g. *Yersinia* enteritis[58]) and its localization. Changes of bowel function can be assessed by measuring SeHCAT retention, vitamin B_{12} absorption, or intestinal permeability (^{51}Cr-EDTA). Using these methods Mahlstedt and coworkers were able to document the clinical course of bowel irritation during and following radiation therapy of abdominal malignomas[59]. In patients presenting diarrhoea of unknown origin, measurements of SeHCAT retention are useful to screen for ileitis or idiopathic bile acid loss[31].

CONCLUSION

The majority of inflammatory bowel diseases can be accurately diagnosed by endoscopy including histology. Therefore only in selected cases will leukocyte scanning for confirming and localizing inflammatory bowel disease be necessary. Seriously ill patients, but also patients suffering from bowel resection or long-lasting inflammation may profit from leukocyte scanning[60], which is the method of choice for proving or excluding inflammation. Additional faecal counting gives a quantitative assessment of disease activity.

Measurement of SeHCAT retention is a simple and non-invasive procedure. It should be used in the follow-up of patients with ileal disease. It may be regarded as the procedure of choice for excluding changes of bowel function in inflammatory ileal disease. Measurement of vitamin B_{12} absorption is less sensitive and should be employed, if ^{14}C-glycocholic acid or the H_2-breath test are not available to prove bacterial overgrowth of the upper intestinal tract. The relevance of testing intestinal permeability is subject to recent work[36]. It may gain importance because of its simple rapid handling. Table 1.6 finally illustrates the indications for nuclear procedures in inflammatory bowel diseases.

Table 1.6 Indications for nuclear diagnostic procedures in inflammatory bowel disease

Test	*Crohn's disease*	*Ulcerative colitis*	*Other*
Leukocyte scanning	++	++	++
Faecal leukocyte excretion	+	+	(+)
SeHCAT retention	+++	+	++
Vitamin B_{12} absorption	++	(+)	+
Intestinal permeability	+	(+)	+
Protein exudation	(+)	(+)	(+)

Test is: +++, highly important and suitable; ++, important but replaceable by other procedures; +, suitable and may yield additional information; (+), suitable in certain situations.

REFERENCES

1. McAffee, J.G. and Thakur, M.L. (1976). Survey of radioactive agents for *in vivo* labelling of phagocytic leukocytes. I. Soluble agents. *J. Nucl. Med.*, **17**, 480–7
2. McAffee, J.G. and Thakur, M.L. (1987). Survey of radioactive agents for *in vivo* labelling of phagocytic leukocytes. II. Particles. *J. Nucl. Med.*, **17**, 488–92
3. Thakur, M.L., Coleman, R.E., Mayhall, C.G. and Welch, M.J. (1976). Preparation and evaluation of In-111 labelled leukocytes as an abscess imaging agent in dogs. *Radiology*, **119**, 731–2
4. Thakur, M.L., Lavender, J.P. and Arnot, R.N. (1977). Indium-111 labelled autologous leukocytes in man. *J. Nucl. Med.*, **18**, 1012–19
5. Becker, W., Fischbach, W., Reiners, C. and Börner, W. (1985). ^{111}In-Oxin markierte Leukozyten: Eine Methode zur Lokalisationsdiagnostik und Aktivitätsbeurteilung von Morbus Crohn und Colitis ulcerosa. *Z. Gastroenterol.*, **23**, 557–64
6. Saverymuttu, S.H., Peters, A.M., Hodgson, H.J. and Chadwick, V.S. (1983). Assessment of disease activity in ulcerative colitis using 111-indium labelled leukocyte faecal excretion. *Scand. J. Gastroenterol.*, **18**, 907–12

7. Paul, J.L., Moissan, A., Cardin, U.L., Le Cloirec, J., Herry, J.H. and Launoise, B. (1985). Recherche des collections suppuries intra-abdominales. *Presse Med.*, **29**, 1367–70
8. Saverymuttu, S.H., Crofton, M.E., Peters, A.M. and Lavender, J.P. (1983). Indium-111 tropolonate leukocyte scanning in the detection of intraabdominal abscesses. *Clin. Radiol.*, **34**, 593–6
9. Becker, W., Fischbach, W., Reiners, C. and Börner, W. (1985). ^{111}In-Oxin markierte Granulozyten bei Morbus Crohn und Colitis ulcerosa – Markierungs- und Untersuchungstechnik. *RöFo*, **142**, 320–5
10. Saverymuttu, S.H., Peters, A.M., Crofton, M.E., Rees, H., Lavender, J.P., Hodgson, H.J. and Chadwick, V.S. (1985). 111-Indium autologous granulocytes in the detection of inflammatory bowel disease. *Gut*, **26**, 955–60
11. Becker, W., Schomann, E., Fischbach, W., Börner, W. and Gruner, K.R. (1988). Comparison of ^{99m}Tc HMPAO and ^{111}In-oxine labelled granulocytes in man: first clinical results. *Nucl. Med. Commun.*, **9**, 435–47
12. Joseph, J., Höffken, H., Bosslet, K. and Schorlemmer, H.U. (1988). *In vivo* labelling of granulocytes with ^{99m}Tc anti-NCA monoclonal antibodies for imaging inflammation. *Eur. J. Nucl. Med.*, **7/8**, 367–73
13. Kroiss, A., Weiss, W., Kölbl, Ch., Dinstl, K. and Neumayr, A. (1988). Neue diagnostische Möglichkeiten bei M. Crohn und Colitis ulcerosa mit 123-J markierten anti-Granulozyten Antikörpern. *Nucl. Med.*, **2**, 19
14. Sfakianakis, G.N., Al-Seikh, W., Heal, A., Rodman, G., Zeppa, R. and Serafini, A. (1982). Comparison of scintigraphy with In-111 leukocytes and ^{67}Ga in the diagnosis of occult sepsis. *J. Nucl. Med.*, **23**, 618–26
15. Kadir, S. and Strauss, H.W. (1976). Evaluation of inflammatory bowel disease with ^{99m}Tc DTPA. *Radiology*, **130**, 443–6
16. Abdel-Dayem, H.M., Mahajan, K.K., Ericsson, S.B.S., Kouris, K., Owunwanne, A., Nawaz, K., Higazi, E. and Awdeh, M. (1986). ^{99m}Tc-DTPA uptake in malignant and inflammatory bowel disease: experience from intestinal bleeding studies. *Nucl. Med. Commun.*, 7, 381–9
17. Dawson, D.J., Khan, A.N., Nutall, P. and Shreeve, D.R. (1985). Technetium-99m labelled sucralphate isotope scanning in the detection of peptic ulceration. *Nucl. Med. Commun.*, **6**, 319–25
18. Vasquez, T.E., Bridges, R.L., Braunstein, P., Jansholt, A.L. and Meshkinpour, H. (1983). Gastrointestinal ulcerations: detection using a technetium-99m-labelled ulcer-avid agent. *Radiology*, **148**, 227–31
19. Crama-Bohbouth, G.E., Arndt, J.W., Pena, A.S., Blok, D., Verspaget, H.W., Weterman, I.T., Lamers, C.B.H.W. and Pauwels, E.K.J. (1988). Is radiolabelled sucralphate scintigraphy of any use in the diagnosis of inflammatory bowel disease? *Nucl. Med. Commun.*, **9**, 591–5
20. Khan, A.N., Miller, V., Ratcliffe, J.F. and Dawson, D.J. (1985). Technetium-99m-sucralphate isotope scanning in the detection of active inflammatory bowel disease in children. *Eur. J. Nucl. Med.*, **2/3**, A33
21. Christian, P.E., Datz, F.L., Sorensen, J.A. and Taylor, A. (1983). Technical factors in gastric emptying studies: teaching editorial. *J. Nucl. Med.*, **3**, 264–8
22. Malagelada, J.R., Robertson, J.S., Brown, M.L., Remington, M., Duenes, J.A., Thornforde, G.M. and Carryer, P.W. (1984). Intestinal transit of solid and liquid components of a meal in health. *Gastroenterology*, **87**, 1255–63
23. Grill, B.B., Lange, R., Markowitz, R., Craig Hillemeier, A., McCallum, R.W. and Gryboski, J.D. (1985). Delayed gastric emptying in children with Crohn's disease. *J. Clin. Gastroenterol.*, **7**, 216–26
24. Lorenz-Meyer, H. and Brandes, W. (1981). Klinik des Morbus Crohn. *Internist*, **22**, 420–9
25. Mekhjian, H.S., Switz, D.M., Melnyk, C.S., Rankin, G.B. and Brooks, R.K. (1979). Clinical features and natural history of Crohn's disease. *Gastroenterology*, **77**, 898–906
26. Rankin, J.B., Watts, H.D., Melnyk, C.S. and Kelley, M.L. (1979). National co-operative Crohn's disease study: extraintestinal manifestations and perianal complications. *Gastroenterology*, **77**, 914–20

27. Agnew, J.E., Pocock, D.G. and Jewell, D.P. (1982). Sacroiliac joint ratios in inflammatory bowel disease: relationship to backpain and to activity of bowel disease. *Br. J. Radiol.*, **55**, 821–6
28. Boyd, G.S., Merrick, M.V., Monks, R. and Thomas, I.L. (1981). Se-75 labelled bile acid analogs, new radiopharmaceuticals for investigating the enterohepatic circulation. *J. Nucl. Med.*, **22**, 720–5
29. Freundlieb, O., Szy, D., Balzer, K. and Strötges, M.W. (1983). Vergleichende Untersuchung über verschiedene Mebverfahren zur Beurteilung der Gallensäureausscheigung mitteis 75-Selen markierter Homotaurocholsäure (75-SeHCAT). *Nucl. Med.*, **5**, 258–61
30. Holdstock, G., Phillips, G., Hames, T.K., Condon, B.R., Fleming, J.S., Smith, C.L. and Ackery, D.M. (1985). Potential of SeHCAT retention as an indicator of terminal ileal involvement in inflammatory bowel disease. *Eur. J. Nucl. Med.*, **10**, 528–30
31. Merrick, M.V., Eastwood, M.A. and Ford, M.J. (1985). Is bile acid malabsorption underdiagnosed? An evaluation of accuracy of diagnosis by measurement of SeHCAT retention. *Br. Med. J.*, No. 6469, 665–8
32. Schilling, R.F. (1953). Intrinsic factor studies. *J. Lab. Clin. Med.*, **42**, 860–8
33. Lindstedt, S. (1957). The turnover of cholic acid in man. *Act. Physiol. Scand.*, **40**, 1–9
34. Hepner, G.W. (1975). Increased sensitivity of the cholyglycine breath test for detecting ileal dysfunction. *Gastroenterology*, **68**, 8–16
35. Fromm, H., Thomas, P.J. and Hofmann, A.F. (1973). Sensitivity and specificity in tests of distal ileal function: prospective comparison of bile acid and vitamin B12 absorption in ileal resection patients. *Gastroenterology*, **64**, 1077–90
36. Bjarnason, J., O'Morain, C., Levi, A.J. and Peters, T.J. (1983). Absorption of 51-chromium labelled ethylenediamine tetraacetate in inflammatory bowel disease. *Gastroenterology*, **85**, 318–22
37. Bjarnason, J., Smethurst, P., Levi, A.J. and Peters, T.J. (1985). Intestinal permeability of ^{51}Cr-EDTA in rats with experimentally induced enteropathy. *Gut*, **26**, 579–85
38. Gordon, R.S. (1959). Exudative enteropathy: abnormal permeability of the gastrointestinal tract demonstrable with labelled polyvinylpyrrolidone. *Lancet*, **1**, 325–6
39. Laster, L., Waldmann, T.A., Fenster, L.F. and Singleton, J.W. (1966). Albumin metabolism in patients with Whipple's disease. *J. Clin. Invest.*, **45**, 637–44
40. Goldberg, H.J., Caruthers Jr., S.B., Nelson, J.A. and Singleton, J.W. (1979). Radiographic findings of the national cooperative Crohn's disease study. *Gastroenterology*, **77**, 925–37
41. Becker, W., Fischbach, W., Reiners, C. and Börner, W. (1986). Three-phase white blood cell scan: diagnostic validity in abdominal inflammatory diseases. *J. Nucl. Med.*, **27**, 1109–15
42. Saverymuttu, S.H., Peters, A.M., Hodgson, H.J., Chadwick, V.S. and Lavender, J.P. (1983). 111-Indium leukocyte scanning in small bowel Crohn's disease. *Gastrointest. Radiol.*, **8**, 157–61
43. Saverymuttu, S.H., Hodgson, H.J. and Chadwick, V.S. (1985). Controlled trial comparing prednisolone with an elemental diet plus non-absorbable antibiotics in active Crohn's disease. *Gut*, **26**, 994–8
44. Stein, D.T., Gray, G.M., Gregory, P.B., Anderson, M., Goodwin, D.A. and Ross McDougall, I. (1983). Location and activity of ulcerative and Crohn's colitis by indium-111 leukocyte scan. *Gastroenterology*, **94**, 388–93
45. Ybern, A., Martin-Cornin, H., Gine, J.J., Casanovas, T., Villa, R. and Gassull, M.A. (1986). 111-In-oxine labelled autologous leukocytes in inflammatory bowel disease: a new scintigraphic activity index. *Eur. J. Nucl. Med.*, **111**, 341–4
46. Best, W.R., Bectel, J.M., Singleton, J.W. and Kern, F. (1976). Development of a Crohn's disease activity index. National co-operative Crohn's disease study. *Gastroenterology*, **70**, 439–44
47. Best, W.R., Bectel, J.M. and Singleton, J.W. (1979). Rederived values of the eight coefficients of the Crohn's disease activity index (CDAI). *Gastroenterology*, **77**, 843–6
48. Saverymuttu, S.H., Lavender, J.P., Hodgson, H.J. and Chadwick, V.S. (1983). Assessment of disease activity in inflammatory bowel disease: a new approach using 111-indium granulocyte scanning. *Br. Med. J.*, **287**, 1751–3

49. Scheurien, C., Kruis, W., Moser, E. and Paumgartner, G. (1988). Accuracy of whole body retention half-life of 75-SeHCAT in the diagnosis of ileal dysfunction in patients with Crohn's disease. *Hepato-Gastroenterology*, **35**, 136–9
50. Fagan, C.A., Chadwick, V.S. and McLean Baird, J. (1983). SeHCAT absorption: A simple test of ileal dysfunction. *Digestion*, **26**, 159–65
51. Nyhlin, H., Merrick, M.V., Eastwood, M.A. and Brydon, W.G. (1983). Evaluation of ileal function using 23-selena-25-homotaurocholate, a gamma-labelled conjugated bile acid – clinical assessment. *Gastroenterology*, **84**, 63–8
52. Thaysen, E.H., Orholm, M., Amfred, T., Carl, J. and Rödbro, P. (1982). Assessment of ileal function by abdominal counting of the retention of a gamma emitting bile acid analogue. *Gut*, **23**, 862–5
53. Knockel, J.Q., Koehler, P.R., Lee, T.G. and Welch, J.M. (1980). Diagnosis of abdominal abscesses with computed tomography, ultrasound and ^{111}In leukocyte scans. *Radiology*, **137**, 425–32
54. Krestin, G.P., Beyer, D. and Steinbrich, W. (1984). Rationelles Vorgehen bei der Diagnostik abdomineller Abszesse mit Hilfe bildgebender Verfahren. *RöFö*, **141**, 673–7
55. Lane, I.F., Poskitt, K., Irwin, J.T.C., Sinclair, M., Jewkes, R.I. and McCollum, C.N. (1985). Abscess diagnosis using ^{111}In leukocytes. *Eur. J. Nucl. Med.*, **2/3**, A26
56. Farivar, S., Fromm, H., Schindler, D., McJunkin, B. and Schmidt, F.W. (1980). Tests of bile acid and vitamin B_{12} metabolism in ileal Crohn's disease. *Am. J. Clin. Pathol.*, **73**, 69–74
57. Holmquist, L., Anderssen, H., Rudic, N., Ahren, C. and Fällström, S.P. (1986). Bile acid malabsorption in children and adolescents with chronic colitis. *Scand. J. Gastroenterol.*, **21**, 87–92
58. Becker, W., Fischbach, W. and Börner, W. (1985). Autologous ^{111}In-oxine labelled granulocytes in *Yersinia* infections. *Eur. J. Nucl. Med.*, **10**, 377–8
59. Mahlstedt, J., Habe, A., Wolf, F., Reichert, M., Duering, A., Herbst, M. and Stoll, R. (1985). Evaluation of small bowel injury after radiotherapy by radioisotopic test. *Nucl. Med. Commun.*, **6**, 601–2
60. Singleton, J.W. and Klingensmith III, W.C. Editorial (1983). Indium-111 leukocyte imaging study in inflammatory bowel disease. *Gastroenterology*, **2**, 426–7

2
Clinical pharmacology of mesalazine (5-aminosalicylic acid) in chronic inflammatory bowel disease

U. KLOTZ

INTRODUCTION

Several new salicylate compounds have been developed in recent years as a result of intensive clinical research with sulphasalazine (SZ). Since its discovery in 1941 SZ has been used as a kind of standard drug in the treatment of chronic inflammatory bowel disease (IBD); especial benefit has been obtained in the management of ulcerative colitis patients. However, therapy with this azo-compound is often limited by dose-dependent side effects and intolerance (for review see references 1 and 2). The mode of action of SZ is still unknown but metabolic and clinical studies have raised the question of whether it is the entire molecule or a metabolite that is the therapeutic principal. In the first controlled clinical trials it was realized that 5-aminosalicylic acid, a major primary metabolite of SZ (now renamed mesalazine) represents the active therapeutic moiety[3–5]. During the last few years these initial studies have been confirmed by numerous investigations and clinical experience with mesalazine has been accumulating. Nowadays this salicylate has a well-established place in the treatment of IBD, especially for such patients as are sensitive to SZ[6–9].

NEW SALICYLATE PREPARATIONS

It seems that mesalazine exerts its therapeutic action mainly from the luminal site of the small and/or large bowel. In addition, most of SZ's side effects can be attributed to the sulphapyridine part of the molecule. These perceptions have been the basis on which new salicylate preparations have been developed and which can be divided into four groups:

(1) conjugated azo-analogues of SZ, in which the 'toxic' sulphapyridine is replaced by an 'inert' carrier as in the case of balsalazide or ipsalazide.

Since these compounds are still in a very early stage of clinical evaluation, they will not be considered further;

(2) special galenic forms of mesalazine designed to 'target' the drug to its proposed site of action; several products are now available in the form of suppositories, enemas and oral formulations;

(3) olsalazine, formerly called azodisalicylate, which consists of two 5-aminosalicylate residues linked by an azo bond;

(4) 4-aminosalicylic acid, well-known as *p*-aminosalicylate (PAS) which is currently under clinical investigation, since its clinical efficacy in ulcerative colitis appears to be similar to that of mesalazine[10].

PHARMACOKINETIC CHARACTERISTICS OF MESALAZINE

Parenteral administration

This route of administration has been selected for research reasons only in order to determine unequivocally the pharmacokinetics of mesalazine. Following a single intravenous infusion of 0.5 g of mesalazine to six healthy women (between 44 and 58 years of age) 53% of the dose could be recovered in the urine over 48 h as acetylated 5-aminosalicylate and 26% as unchanged drug. Elimination of mesalazine is rapid – as characterized by a short elimination half-life ($t_{1/2}$) of 42 min and a total plasma clearance (CL) of 300 ml min^{-1}. The apparent volume of distribution averaged 18 L. Elimination of the major metabolite was slower (apparent $t_{1/2}$ = 78 min; CL = 217 ml min^{-1}). Initial plasma concentrations of mesalazine were high (50.5 ± 12.5 μg ml^{-1}) but 7 h after the infusion almost no drug and metabolite were measurable[11].

Oral administration

After oral intake of mesalazine in uncoated form the compound will be absorbed rapidly and to a large extent already in the stomach. Urinary excretion of mesalazine and its acetylated metabolite averaged 21 and 31% of the dose, respectively. The bioavailability calculated from areas under the serum concentration curves was 75%[11].

Coating of mesalazine with the acrylic polymer Eudragit S (Asacol) resulted in a reduced absorption since only 3 and 18% of a single dose could be recovered as mesalazine or acetylated metabolite, respectively, in the urine. Both agents were slightly more slowly eliminated ($t_{1/2}$ 67 min and 137 min, respectively) than following intravenous administration[11]. In patients with ulcerative colitis, considerable variation in the individual plasma concentration–time profiles were noted which was due to the different disintegration times of the tablets[12].

In Pentasa, mesalazine is microencapsulated in ethylcellulose beads which release the drug throughout the intestinal tract and about 53% (12% as unchanged drug; 41% as acetylated metabolite) and 40% (14% as mesalazine; 26% as metabolite) of the dose could be recovered in urine or faeces, respectively. In 14 healthy volunteers on 1500 mg mesalazine per day the steady state plasma levels of acetylated mesalazine ranged[13] between 1.1 and 2.9 $\mu g\ ml^{-1}$.

In Salofalk, (and the identical Claversal) 5-aminosalicylate is coated with another acrylic polymer (Eudragit L) and with cellulose ether. The controlled release preparation is additionally buffered with sodium carbonate and glycine. These formulations release mesalazine in the terminal ileum and into the large bowel. Urinary (11% mesalazine; 33% metabolite) and fecal (16% mesalazine; 19% metabolite) recoveries indicate some absorption as well as intestinal availability[14]. If these preparations were labelled with ^{111}indium it could be visualized that disintegration of most tablets took place 3.2 h after emptying of the stomach into the small intestine and approximately 80% of doses resulted in drug dispersion within the ascending colon[15,16]. Following a single oral dose of 500 mg, mesalazine and its metabolite could first be detected in plasma after 5 h and maximal plasma levels of between 0.5 and 1.5 $\mu g\ ml^{-1}$ were reached after approximately 7 h[17]. Similarly, at steady state (500 mg tid) peak levels (1–2 $\mu g\ ml^{-1}$) were observed, following a lag time of 3 to 4 h, after about 6 h. Under both dosage regimens $t_{1/2}$ was around 1.4 h[14,17].

In a recent crossover study, in eight healthy volunteers, these three oral formulations were directly compared by measuring urinary and fecal excretion and no significant differences between Pentasa, Asacol and Salofalk were recorded[18]. Likewise, with all mesalazine preparations plasma concentrations were similar (range 0.02–2.9 $\mu g\ ml^{-1}$. The acetylated metabolite concentrations always exceeded those of the parent drug by a factor of one and a half to three[19].

Coating mesalazine prevents release of the drug in the stomach or at an acidic pH value. Release depends mainly on the intestinal pH and partly also on gastrointestinal transit time. Most of the drug is delivered more proximally and continuously into the colon. Thus, the therapeutic success of 'targeted' delivery to specific sites of inflammation depends upon the release pattern of the formulation, the individual site of inflammation, pH and transit time. These factors are likely to vary from patient to patient much more than the minor differences between the three different preparations.

When normal intestinal transit time (16–26 h) was accelerated (to 4–9 h) in seven healthy volunteers by a laxative, fecal excretion of total mesalazine increased from 16 to 29%, which was associated with a corresponding decline in urinary excretion from 32 to 21%. Thus, the Pentasa preparation used still released sufficient mesalazine[20].

Rectal administration

From enemas containing 700 mg 5-aminosalicylate and 300 mg xanthan hydrophilic gum, only 2–11% of the dose could be recovered in the urine during 8 h after administration – indicating poor absorption in patients with ulcerative colitis[21]. Dependent on the pH value of the solvent used for another enema preparation, plasma concentrations of 5-aminosalicylate and of its acetylated metabolite were two to three times higher following the neutral solution than if citrate buffer of pH 4.8 was used. Only the metabolite could be recovered in the urine (35 *vs* 21%) whereas unchanged mesalazine (26 *vs* 44% recovery) dominated in the faeces[22]. If the neutral solution of mesalazine (500 mg) was instilled into the right part of the colon or the rectum of six healthy subjects, urinary excretion of total 5-aminosalicylate averaged 25 and 33% of the dose, respectively. Plasma levels of the metabolite (1.3–2.2 μg ml^{-1}) were considerably higher than those of mesalazine (0.2–0.6 μg ml^{-1}). These results indicate that absorption of mesalazine is pH-dependent but similar in the right and the left parts of the colon[23].

In addition to enemas, suppositories of mesalazine are used mainly for the treatment of ulcerative colitis and proctitis. In one clinical study 7–51% of the daily dose could be recovered in acetylated form in the 24-h urine of patients with proctitis[4]. From Salofalk suppositories, on average 13% of the maintenance dose of 1.5 g per day was recovered in the urine of patients with ulcerative colitis. Steady state concentrations of mesalazine (0.1 μg ml^{-1}) and acetylated metabolite (0.5 μg ml^{-1}) were relatively low[24].

Other pharmakokinetic properties of mesalazine

The plasma protein-binding of mesalazine (43%) and its acetylated metabolite (78–83%) will not restrict the elimination or distribution of either agent[14,25].

Since only a limited fraction of mesalazine is absorbed its penetration into the milk of nursing mothers can be neglected; in the form of the metabolite, 0.1% of the administered dose were excreted by this route[26]. Similarly, biliary excretion of mesalazine (mainly in conjugated form) is low (<1% of administered dose) and consequently only minor enterohepatic recycling can be assumed[24,27].

Mesalazine is mainly excreted in acetylated form into the urine. It is not therefore surprising that this major metabolite will accumulate in patients with renal failure undergoing haemodialysis. During a dialysis period of 4 h (flow rate 200 ml min^{-1}) the initially high plasma levels of acetylated 5-aminosalicylate (dose-dependent range 34–118 μg ml^{-1}) fall to 13–30 μg ml^{-1}. Extraction ratio (0.3–0.5) and dialysance (60–100 ml min^{-1}) indicate a very effective removal by haemodialysis[28].

Based on steady-state plasma level monitoring and urinary excretion data in pediatric patients, there appears to be no significant difference in the disposition of mesalazine between children (age range 2–16 years) and adults[19,29]. In Table 2.1 the most important pharmacokinetic parameters of mesalazine are summarized.

Table 2.1 Pharmacokinetic properties of mesalazine

(1)	Fast elimination by acetylation ($t_{1/2}$: 0.5–2 h; CL = 300 ml min^{-1})	
(2)	Relative low volume of distribution and plasma protein-binding (V = 18 L; f_u = 57%)	
(3)	Extent of absorption dependent on galenic formulation:	
	suppositories	10–15%
	enemas	10–25%
	oral controlled release	20–50%
(4)	Low steady-state plasma levels	
	5-AS:	0.02–2 μg ml^{-1}
	Ac-5-AS:	0.1–3 μg ml^{-1}

METABOLISM OF MESALAZINE

As already described, the absorbed mesalazine is mainly excreted as acetylated salicylate into the urine. This metabolic step is independent of the acetylator status[30] and not reversible[31,32]. It takes place during the first passage of mesalazine through the intestinal mucosa and liver[33] and both acetylation processes are probably saturable[30]. While acetylation by fecal bacteria can be neglected[17], there appears to be early intraluminal acetylation, since the metabolite could be detected in the juice of the small bowel[34]. The extensive presystemic and preabsorptive acetylation is responsible for the fast elimination of mesalazine ($t_{1/2}$ = 0.5–2.4 h) and its low bioavailability. Since the acetylated metabolite is eliminated much more slowly than the mesalazine[32,35], with an apparent $t_{1/2}$ of 6–12 h and a renal CL between 200 and 400 ml min^{-1}, its plasma levels always exceed those of the parent compound.

PHARMACOKINETIC CHARACTERISTICS OF OLSALAZINE

The azo-bond of this prodrug has to be split by colonic bacteria before mesalazine can exert its action. Less than 5% of an oral dose was excreted unchanged in the urine (renal CL 1.6–2.8 ml min^{-1}). Dose-dependent steady-state plasma levels of olsalazine (e.g. 4–12 μg ml^{-1} with 2 g per day) are reached within 6 to 28 days, due to a long $t_{1/2}$ between 4 and 13 days. Serum concentration of mesalazine (undetectable to 0.8 μg ml^{-1}) and its acetylated metabolite (1.1 μg ml^{-1}) were much lower. Between 6 and 25% of a daily dose are excreted in the urine, predominantly as acetylated 5-aminosalicylate. Fecal recovery of mesalazine and its metabolite ranged from 13 to 30% and from 20 to 55% respectively[36,37]. Following a single oral dose of olsalazine (500 mg) in healthy volunteers, cumulative excretion (96 h) of total salicylates with urine and faeces was about 25 and 47%, respectively[18].

Recently an intravenous dose of 10 mg olsalazine was administered to seven healthy male volunteers and a much shorter $t_{1/2}$ of 0.9±0.6 h and a higher CL of 83 ml min^{-1} were calculated. The extensive plasma protein-binding of olsalazine (99.8%) results in a relatively small distribution volume (5 L). The discrepancy in elimination rate is most likely due to the fact that in the two previous studies olsalazine and its sulphate conjugate have been codetermined[38].

THERAPEUTIC VALUE OF MESALAZINE

From numerous controlled clinical trials, there is accumulating evidence that mesalazine, whether administered rectally or orally, is effective in the treatment of acute IBD. With doses between 0.4 and 4 g per day, remission rates in patients with ulcerative colitis of about 75% could be observed (for review see references 7, 9 and 39).

This general impression has been confirmed by several more recent studies. While in patients with active Crohn's disease in the small bowel, a treatment period of 16 weeks with oral mesalazine (Pentasa 1500 mg per day) was only slightly more effective than placebo[40], a higher oral dosage (Asacol 4.8 g per day) was clearly superior ($p < 0.0001$) to placebo in patients with active ulcerative colitis[41]. Another prospective open study reported, after a 4-week treatment with 3.2 g per day, a remission rate of 64% in patients with mild to moderate active ulcerative colitis[42]. In a 4-week trial with oral mesalazine (2.4 g per day) symptomatic remission was seen in 43% of patients with ulcerative colitis[43].

Complete clinical remission could be induced in 56% of patients with idiopathic proctitis by treatment with suppositories (300 mg bid) of mesalazine[44]. Enemas of mesalazine have been used with great success in patients with distal ulcerative colitis and proctitis. After treatment for 4 or 6 weeks, remission rates of 70 and 63% have been observed in different trials[45,46].

Drug treatment of IBD should also prevent a relapse of the chronic disease. Literature data indicate that mesalazine is probably also valuable for such prophylactic treatment (for review see reference 39). Recently, in patients with ulcerative colitis relapse rates of 37.5% have been reported during a 48-week treatment with oral mesalazine (Asacol, 0.8–1.2 mg per day). Comparative data[47] for the sulphasalazine group (2–3 g per day) were 38.6%. A sustained clinical and endoscopic remission upon 1 year follow-up of 78% could be observed in 50 patients with ulcerative colitis treated orally with 800 mg four times daily[42].

Likewise, a relapse rate of 17% was observed within 9 months in patients with distal ulcerative colitis and proctitis when treated with enemas (2 or 4 g) of mesalazine[48]. When a lower dose (1 g per day) was used annual relapse rate in patients with left-sided ulcerative colitis was 25% with mesalazine but 85% with placebo[49].

Sufficient solid clinical data are now available which prove that mesalazine is at least as effective as the standard drug SZ in the treatment of IBD, especially ulcerative colitis (see also Table 2.2). In some comparative studies mesalazine was even slightly superior to SZ. However, the major advantage of mesalazine, which represents a progress in drug treatment of IBD, is the improved tolerance to this 'new' drug or 'old' active metabolite. Whereas treatment with SZ has to be stopped in at least 10 to 20% of patients because of dose-dependent side effects or unwanted drug reactions, mesalazine is well tolerated by most patients, and in contrast to SZ there are no fertility problems with mesalazine. In numerous crossover trials among SZ-sensitive patients showing intolerance or allergic reactions to this sulphapyridine-containing azo-compound only about 10% of those subjects showed similar reactions to the new mesalazine preparations (for review see references 39, 50 and 51).

Table 2.2 Clinical efficacy of mesalazine in IBD

Induction of remission in acute attacks

Rectal treatment of ulcerative colitis/proctitis:
remission rate between 56 and 85%

Oral treatment of IBD:
remission rate between 43 and 85%

Prevention of relapse

Annual relapse rate in ulcerative colitis:
with oral treatment 22–38%
with enemas 25%

In contrast to other salicylates, mesalazine had no effect on platelet aggregation and fibrinolytic activity[52]. With the enemas some anal canal irritations can occur but seldom[49]. Several rare adverse events to mesalazine have been reported: mainly nausea, abdominal discomfort, headache, exacerbation of disease state, reversible mild neutropenia, transient elevation of liver enzyme values, fever or retrosternal chest pain[42,50,51]. In summarizing all clinical studies with mesalazine, less than 5% of patients reported side effects.

Acute animal experiments with high intravenous dosing of 5-aminosalicylate give some concern about nephrotoxicity. However, when kidney function was thoroughly monitored in the clinical trials no impairment in kidney function was observed[47,48,53,54]. So far two patients on mesalazine (2.4 g daily) developed minor rises in plasma creatinine (up to twofold); both resolved spontaneously. Neither patient had abnormalities on urine testing[43]. Since experience with high doses of mesalazine is still somewhat limited, it appears prudent to control kidney function especially during long-term treatment (see also Table 2.3).

THERAPEUTIC VALUE OF OLSALAZINE

There are some studies indicating that oral olsalazine is effective in the treatment of acute ulcerative colitis[55,56] and in preventing a relapse[57]. However, in two other studies no significant difference in clinical improvement in patients with ulcerative colitis between olsalazine enemas (1 g per day) or capsules (1 g bid) and placebo was reported[56,58].

Table 2.3 Safety aspects for mesalazine

Lower incidence of (allergic) intolerance compared to SZ (about ten fold)
No fertility problems in males (in contrast to SZ)
No effect on platelet aggregation and fibrinolytic activity (in contrast to other salicylates)
No induction of diarrhoea (in contrast to olsalazine)
Low incidence of adverse reaction (≤5%), mainly nausea, abdominal discomfort, headache, exacerbation of disease, fever, retrosternal chest pain
No nephrotoxicity, but kidney function should be controlled during long-term treatment with high doses

In general, the spectrum of side effects of olsalazine is similar to that of mesalazine. There is a striking difference between the agents where gastrointestinal symptoms are concerned. The new prodrug olsalazine induces in at least 10–15% of patients, diarrhoea or loose stools[56–58]. In other clinical studies, higher percentages of 35%[59] or even 76%[60] were observed. This high incidence will limit the utility of olsalazine. The side effect can already be seen about 4 h after single oral doses in healthy subjects and it is probably dose-dependent[38]: 25% diarrhoea with 1 g, 100% diarrhoea with 4 g.

PROPOSED MODE OF ACTION OF MESALAZINE

Based mainly on biochemical *in vitro* experiments, several working hypotheses have been popular. Since prostaglandins and leukotrienes are involved in inflammatory processes, the inhibition of the lipoxygenase pathway[59,61] and leukotriene formation by 5-aminosalicylate[62] could be one possibility.

It has been shown that mesalazine in the presence of nitrite inhibits β-oxidation of short-chain fatty acids in isolated colonic epithelial cells. Whether this has implications both for the pathogenesis of IBD and the therapeutic action of mesalazine remains to be elucidated[63].

Another working hypothesis has concentrated on the oxygen-radical scavenging properties of 5-aminosalicylate. Since reactive oxygen species can cause inflammation and 5-aminosalicylate (in a remarkably dose-related manner) suppressed the production of $OH^{\cdot}$ this may at least partly explain the therapeutic efficacy of mesalazine[64–66].

Independent of the molecular mechanism of mesalazine's action there is also some discussion as to whether acetylated 5-aminosalicylate will contribute[67] to clinical efficacy or is inactive[44,68].

CONCLUSIONS

The pharmacokinetic properties and clinical characteristics of mesalazine have been characterized comprehensively in many studies. It seems to be important that sufficient amounts of active drug are available at the luminal site of the gastrointestinal tract and/or in the inflamed mucosa cells. For many patients intolerant to SZ or suffering from its numerous side effects, mesalazine has proven to be a very valuable alternative. Its clinical efficacy in IBD and the favourable low incidence of side effects is documented in numerous controlled clinical studies; mesalazine has made a significant contribution to progress in the treatment of IBD.

ACKNOWLEDGEMENT

This work was supported by the Robert Bosch Foundation (Stuttgart, FRG). I am indebted to Mrs Grözinger for preparing the manuscript.

REFERENCES

1. Bachrach, W.H. (1988). Sulfasalazine: I. An historical perspective. *Am. J. Gastroenterol.*, **83**, 487–96
2. Peppercorn, N.A. (1984). Sulfasalazine-pharmacology, clinical use, toxicity, and related new drug development. *Ann. Intern. Med.*, **3**, 377–86
3. Azad Khan, K.A., Piris, J. and Truelove, S.C. (1977). An experiment to determine the active therapeutic moiety of sulphasalazine. *Lancet*, **2**, 892–5
4. van Hees, P.A.M., Bakker, J.H. and van Tongeren, J.H.M. (1980). Effect of sulfapyridine, 5-aminosalicylic acid, and placebo in patients with idiopathic proctitis: a study to determine the active therapeutic moiety of sulphasalazine. *Gut*, **21**, 632–5
5. Klotz, U., Maier, K., Fischer, C. and Heinkel, K. (1980). Therapeutic efficacy of sulfasalazine and its metabolites in patients with ulcerative colitis and Crohn's disease. *N. Engl. J. Med.*, **303**, 1499–502
6. Hawkey, C.J. (1986). Salicylates for the sulfa-sensitive patient with ulcerative colitis. *Gastroenterology*, **90**, 1082–4
7. Williams, C.N. (1987). Clinical experience with 5-aminosalicylate preparations in inflammatory bowel disease – a review. *Can. J. Gastroenterol.*, **83**, 64–7
8. Meyer, S. (1988). The place of oral 5-aminosalicylic acid in the therapy of ulcerative colitis. *Am. J. Gastroenterol.*, **83**, 64–7
9. Margolin, M.L., Krumholz, M.P., Fochios, S.E. and Korelitz, B.I. (1988). Clinical trials in ulcerative colitis: II. Historical review. *Am. J. Gastroenterol.*, **83**, 227–43
10. Campieri, M., Lanfranchi, G.A., Brignola, C. *et al.* (1984). A double blind clinical trial to compare the effects of 4-aminosalicylic acid to 5-aminosalicylic acid in topical treatment of ulcerative colitis. *Digestion*, **29**, 478–9

11. Myers, B., Evans, D.N.W., Rhodes, J., Evans, B.K., Hughes, B.R., Lee, M.G., Richens, A. and Richards, D. (1987). Metabolism and urinary excretion of 5-aminosalicylic acid in healthy volunteers when given intravenously or released for absorption at different sites in the gastrointestinal tract. *Gut*, 196–200
12. Dew, M.J., Ryder, R.E.J., Evans, N., Evans, B.K. and Rhodes, J. (1983). Colonic release of 5-aminosalicylic acid from an oral preparation in active ulcerative colitis. *Br. J. Clin. Pharmacol.*, **16**, 185–7
13. Rasmussen, S.N., Bondesen, S., Hvidberg, E.F., Hansen, S.H., Binder, V., Halskov, S. and Flachs, H. (1982). 5-Aminosalicylic acid in slow release preparation: bioavailability, plasma level and excretion in humans. *Gastroenterology*, **83**, 1062–70
14. Klotz, U., Maier, K.E., Fischer, C. and Bauer, K.H. (1985). A new slow-release form of 5-aminosalicylic acid for the oral treatment of inflammatory bowel disease. Biopharmaceutical and clinical pharmacokinetic characteristics. *Arzneim. Forsch.*, **35**, 636–9
15. Hardy, J.G., Healey, J.N.C., Lee, S.W. and Reynolds, J.R. (1987). Gastrointestinal transit of an enteric-coated delayed-release 5-aminosalicylic acid tablet. *Aliment. Pharmacol. Ther.*, **1**, 209–16
16. Hardy, J.G., Healey, J.N.C. and Reynolds, J.R. (1987). Evaluation of an enteric-coated delayed release 5-aminosalicylic acid tablet in patients with inflammatory bowel disease. *Aliment. Pharmacol. Ther.*, **1**, 273–80
17. Klotz, U., Seyffer, R., Allgayer, H. and Maier, K.E. (1988). Pharmacokinetic properties of mesalazine (5-aminosalicylic acid). In MacDermott, R.P. (ed.) *Inflammatory Bowel Disease*, pp. 725–9. (Amsterdam: Elsevier Science Publisher)
18. Rijk, M.C.M., van Schaik, A. and van Tongeren, J.H.M. (1988). Disposition of 5-aminosalicylic acid by 5-aminosalicylic acid-delivering compounds. *Scand. J. Gastroenterol.*, **23**, 107–12
19. Bondesen, S., Nielsen, O.H., Schou, J.B., Jensen, P.H., Lassen, L.B., Binder, V., Krasilnikoff, P.A., Dano, P., Hansen, S.H., Rasmussen, S.N. and Hvidberg, E.F. (1986). Steady-state kinetics of 5-aminosalicylic acid and sulfapyridine during sulfasalazine prophylaxis in ulcerative colitis. *Scand. J. Gastroenterol.*, **21**, 693–700
20. Christensen, L.A., Slot, O., Sanchez, G., Boserup, J., Rasmussen, S.N., Bondesen, S., Hansen, S.H. and Hvidberg, E.F. (1987). Release of 5-aminosalicylic acid from Pentasa during normal and accelerated intestinal transit time. *Br. J. Clin. Pharmacol.*, **23**, 365–9
21. Dew, M.J., Cardwell, M., Kidwai, N.S., Evans, B.K. and Rhodes, E.J. (1983). 5-Aminosalicylic acid in serum and urine after administration by enema to patients with colitis. *J. Pharm. Pharmacol.*, **35**, 323–4
22. Bondesen, S., Nielsen, O.H., Jacobsen, O., Rasmussen, S.N., Hansen, S.H., Halskov, S., Binder, V. and Hvidberg, E.F. (1984). 5-Aminosalicylic acid enemas in patients with active ulcerative colitis. *Scand. J. Gastroenterol.*, **19**, 677–82
23. Bondesen, S., Schou, J.B., Pedersen, V., Rafiolsada, Z., Hansen, S.H. and Hvidberg, E.F. (1988). Absorption of 5-aminosalicylic acid from colon and rectum. *Br. J. Clin. Pharmacol.*, **25**, 269–72
24. Fischer, C., Maier, K., Stumpf, E., von Gaisburg, U. and Klotz, U. (1983). Disposition of 5-aminosalicylic acid, the active metabolite of sulphasalazine, in man. *Eur. J. Clin. Pharmacol.*, **25**, 511–5
25. Rasmussen, S.N., Binder, V., Maier, K., Bondesen, S., Fischer, C., Klotz, U., Hansen, S.H. and Hvidberg, E.F. (1983). Treatment of Crohn's disease with peroral 5-aminosalicylic acid. *Gastroenterology*, **85**, 1350–3
26. Klotz, U. (1986). Klinische Pharmakologie von 5-Aminosalicylsäure. In Ewe, K. and Fahrländer, H. (eds.) *Therapie chronisch entzündlicher Darmerkrankungen*, pp. 221–7. (Stuttgart/New York: Schattauer Verlag)
27. Fischer, C., Maier, K. and Klotz, U. (1983). Specific measurements of 5-aminosalicylic acid and its acetylated metabolite in human bile. *Br. J. Clin. Pharmacol.*, **15**, 273–4
28. Klotz, U. (1988). Pharmacokinetic properties of 5-aminosalicylic acid (mesalazine). In Goebell, H., Peskar, B.M. and Malchow, H. (eds.) *Inflammatory bowel disease – basic research and clinical implications*, pp. 339–47. (Lancaster: MTP Press)

29. Tolia, V., Massoud, N. and Klotz, U. (1989). Oral 5-aminosalicylic acid in children with chronic inflammatory bowel disease: clinical and pharmacokinetic experience. *J. Pediatr. Gastroenterol.*, **8**, 333–338
30. Klotz, U. (1985). Clinical pharmacokinetics of sulphasalazine, its metabolites and other prodrugs of 5-aminosalicylic acid. *Clin. Pharmacokinet.*, **10**, 285–302
31. Fischer, C., Meese, C.O. and Klotz, U. (1984). A stable isotope method for the quantification of *N*-acetyl-5-aminosalicylic acid in plasma and urine. *Biomed. Mass Spectrum*, **11**, 539–44
32. Meese, C.O., Fischer, C. and Klotz, U. (1984). Is *N*-acetylation of 5-aminosalicylic acid reversible in man? *Br. J. Clin. Pharmacol.*, **18**, 612–5
33. Allgayer, H., Kruis, W. and Paumgartner, G. (1984). Azetylatorstatusunabhängige *N*-Acetyltransferaseaktivität im Kolon bei Patienten mit colitis ulcerosa unter Sulfasalazin-Dauertherapie. *Z. Gastroenterol.*, **22**, 131
34. Layer, P., Goebell, H., Nehlsen, B. and Klotz, U. (1989). Small intestinal transit and delivery to the distal ileal lumen of oral slow release mesalazine (5-ASA) in humans. *Gastroenterol.*, **96**, A292
35. Shaffer, J.L., Turner, M. and Houston, J.B. (1985). Disposition of 5-aminosalicylic acid preparation in patients with inflammatory bowel disease. *Br. J. Clin. Pharmacol.*, **20**, 532P
36. Willoughby, C.P., Aronson, J.K., Agback, H., Boden, N.O. and Truelove, S.C. (1982). Distribution and metabolism in healthy subjects of disodium azodisalicylate, a potential therapeutic agent for ulcerative colitis. *Gut*, **23**, 1081–7
37. van Hogezand, R.A., van Hees, P.A.M., Zwanenburg, B., van Rossum, J.M. and van Tongeren, J.H.M. (1985). Disposition of disodium azodisalicylate in healthy subjects. *Gastroenterology*, **88**, 17–22
38. Ryde, E.M. and Ahnfelt, N.O. (1988). The pharmacokinetics of olsalazine sodium in healthy volunteers after a single i.v. dose and after oral doses with and without food. *Eur. J. Clin. Pharmacol.*, **34**, 481–8
39. Klotz, U. and Maier, K.E. (1987). Pharmacology and pharmacokinetics of 5-aminosalicylic acid. *Dig. Dis. Sci.*, **32**, 46S–50S
40. Rasmussen, S.N., Lauritsen, K., Tage-Jensen, U., Nielsen, O.H., Bytzer, P., Jacobsen, O., Ladefoged, K., Vilien, M., Bincer, V., Rask-Madsen, J., Bondesen, S., Hansen, S.H. and Hvidberg, E.F. (1987). 5-Aminosalicylic acid in the treatment of Crohn's disease. *Scand. J. Gastroenterol.*, **22**, 877–83
41. Schroeder, K.W., Tremaine, W.J. and Ilstrup, D.M. (1987). Coated oral 5-aminosalicylic acid therapy for mildly to moderately active ulcerative colitis. *N. Engl. J. Med.*, **317**, 1625–9
42. Habal, F.M. and Greenberg, G.R. (1988). Treatment of ulcerative colitis with oral 5-aminosalicylic acid including patients with adverse reactions to sulfasalazine. *Am. J. Gastroenterol.*, **83**, 15–19
43. Riley, S.A., Mani, V., Goodman, M.J., Herd, M.E., Dutt, S. and Turnberg, L.A. (1983). Comparison of delayed release 5-aminosalicylic acid (mesalazine) and sulphasalazine in treatment of mild to moderate ulcerative colitis relapse. *Gut*, **29**, 669–74
44. van Hogezand, R.A., van Hees, P.A.M., van Gorp, J.P.W.M., van Lier, H.J.J., Bakker, J.H., Wesseling, P., van Haelst, U.J.G.M. and van Tongeren, J.H.M. (1988). Double-blind comparison of 5-aminosalicylic acid and acetyl-5-aminosalicylic acid suppositories in patients with idiopathic proctitis. *Aliment. Pharmacol. Ther.*, **2**, 33–40
45. Basilisco, G., Ranzi, T., Campanini, M., Piodi, L., Velio, P. and Bianchi, P.A. (1987). 5-Aminosalicylic acid or sulfasalazine retention enemas in distal ulcerative colitis. *Curr. Ther. Res.*, **42**, 910–5
46. Sutherland, L.R., Martin, F., Greer, S., Robinson, M., Greenberger, N., Saibil, F., Martin, T., Sparr, J., Prokipchuk, E. and Borgen, L. (1987). 5-Aminosalicylic acid enemas in the treatment of distal ulcerative colitis, proctosigmoiditis, and proctitis. *Gastroenterology*, **92**, 1894–8
47. Riley, S.A., Mani, V., Goodman, M.J., Herd, M.E., Dutt, S. and Turnberg, L.A. (1988). Comparison of delayed-release 5-aminosalicylic acid (mesalazine) and sulfasalazine as maintenance treatment for patients with ulcerative colitis. *Gastroenterology*, **94**, 1383–9

48. Sutherland, L.R. and Martin, F. (1987). 5-Aminosalicylic acid enemas in the maintenance of remission in distal ulcerative colitis and proctitis. *Can. J. Gastroenterol.*, **1**, 3–6
49. Biddle, W.L., Greenberger, N.J., Swan, T., McPhee, M.S. and Miner Jr., P.B. (1988). 5-Aminosalicylic acid enemas. Effective agent in maintaining remission in left-sided ulcerative colitis. *Gastroenterology*, **94**, 1075–9
50. Burke, D.A., Manning, A.P., Williamson, J.M.S. and Axon, A.T.R. (1987). Adverse reactions to sulphasalazine and 5-amino salicylic acid in the same patient. *Aliment. Pharmacol. Ther.*, **1**, 201–8
51. Turunen, U., Elomaa, I., Anttila, V-J and Seppälä, K. (1987). Mesalazine tolerance in patients with inflammatory bowel disease and previous intolerance or allergy to sulphasalazine or sulphonamides. *Scand. J. Gastroenterol.*, **22**, 798–802
52. Winter, K., Bondesen, S., Hansen, S.H. and Hvidberg, E.F. (1987). Lack of effect of 5-aminosalicylic acid on platelet aggregation and fibrinolytic activity *in vivo* and *in vitro*. *Eur. J. Clin. Pharmacol.*, **33**, 419–22
53. Diener, U., Tuczek, H.V., Fischer, C., Maier, K. and Klotz, U. (1984). Renal function was not impaired by treatment with 5-aminosalicylic acid in rats and man. *Naunyn-Schmiedeberg's Arch. Pharmacol.*, **326**, 278–82
54. Campieri, M., Brignola, C., Bazzocchi, G., Minguzzi, M.R., Gionchetti, P., Belluzzi, A., Adami, F., Basso, O., Migaldi, M.P. and Lanfranchi, G.A. (1986). Several aspects of topical treatment with 5-aminosalicylic acid enemas. In Ewe, K. and Fahrländer, H. (eds.) *Therapie chronisch entzündlicher Darmerkrankungen-Fortschritte, Entwicklungen, Tendenzen* pp. 237–42. (Stuttgart/New York: Schattauer)
55. Meyers, S., Sachar, D.B., Present, D.H. and Janowitz, H.D. (1987). Olsalazine sodium in the treatment of ulcerative colitis among patients intolerant to sulfasalazine. *Gastroenterology*, **93**, 1255–62
56. Selby, W.S., Barr, G.D., Ireland, A., Mason, C.H. and Jewell, D.P. (1985). Olsalazine in active ulcerative colitis. *Br. Med. J.*, **291**, 1373–5
57. Sandberg-Gertzen, H., Järnerot, G. and Kraaz, W. (1986). Azodisal sodium in the treatment of ulcerative colitis. *Gastroenterology*, **90**, 1024–30
58. Hetzel, D.J., Shearman, D.J.C., Bochner, F., Imhoff, D.M., Gibson, G.E., Fitch, R.J., Hecker, R., Labrooy, J. and Rowland, R. (1986). Azodisalicylate (olsalazine) in the treatment of active ulcerative colitis. A placebo controlled clinical trial and assessment of drug disposition. *J. Gastroenterol. Hepatol.*, **1**, 257–66
59. Lauritsen, K., Laursen, L.S., Bukhave, K. and Rask-Madsen, J. (1988). Longterm olsalazine treatment: pharmacokinetics, tolerance and effects on local eicosanoid formation in ulcerative colitis and Crohn's colitis. *Gut*, **29**, 974–82
60. Robinson, M.G. and Dorrough, C. (1987). Azodisalicylate sodium in the treatment of ulcerative colitis. A randomized double-blind, placebo-controlled clinical trial. *Am. J. Gastroenterol.*, **82**, Abstract 124
61. Stenson, W.F. and Lobos, E. (1982). Sulfasalazine inhibits the synthesis of chemotactic lipids by neutrophils. *J. Clin. Invest.*, **69**, 494–7
62. Peskar, B.M., Dreyling, K.W., Peskar, B.A., May, B. and Goebell, H. (1986). Enhanced formation of sulfidopeptide-leukotrienes in ulcerative colitis and Crohn's disease: inhibition by sulfasalazine and 5-aminosalicylic acid. *Agents Actions*, **18**, 381–3
63. Roediger, W., Schapel, G., Lawson, M., Radcliffe, B. and Nance, S. (1986). Effect of 5-aminosalicylic acid (5-ASA) and other salicylates on short-chain fat metabolism in the colonic mucosa. *Biochem. Pharmacol.*, **35**, 221–5
64. Miyachi, Y., Yoshioka, A., Imamura, S. and Niwa, Y. (1987). Effect of sulphasalazine and its metabolites on the generation of reactive oxygen species. *Gut*, **28**, 190–5
65. Craven, P.A., Pfanstiel, J., Saito, R. and de Rubertis, F.R. (1987). Actions of sulfasalazine and 5-aminosalicylic acid as reactive oxygen scavengers in the suppression of bile acid-induced increases in colonic epithelial cell loss and proliferative activity. *Gastroenterology*, **92**, 1998–2008
66. Kvietys, P.R., Smith, S.M., Grisham, M.B. and Manci, E.A. (1988). 5-Aminosalicylic acid protects against ischemia/reperfusion-induced gastric bleeding in the rat. *Gastroenterology*, **94**, 733–8

67. Willoughby, C.P., Piris, J. and Truelove, S.C. (1980). The effect of topical *N*-acetyl-5-aminosalicylic acid in ulcerative colitis. *Scand. J. Gastroenterol.*, **15**, 715–9
68. Binder, V., Halskov, S., Hvidberg, E., Kristensen, E., Riis, P., Tougaard, L. and Willumsen, L. (1981). A controlled study of 5-acetylaminosalicylic acid (5-ac-ASA) as enema in ulcerative colitis. *Scand. J. Gastroenterol.*, (Abstract), **16**, 1122

3
Conservative treatment of Crohn's disease

H. WIETHOLTZ, H.J. THON, R. BÜCHSEL AND S. MATERN

INTRODUCTION

Crohn's disease is a disease of modern Western civilization; it has experienced a tremendous increase since 1960. Incidence rates in Northern Europe and the United States are now up to 8.8/100 000 inhabitants per year and prevalence rates up to 106/100 000 inhabitants (Table 3.1). Despite very extensive investigation, the aetiology of Crohn's disease remains unknown and, in consequence, to date no causal therapy exists. Thus Dr Crohn's statement made in 1932 is still valid and true: 'Medical treatment is purely palliative and supportive'[1].

Major determinants of treatment are activity, as assessed by the activity indices proposed by Best[12], Van Hees[13] or Harvey[14], and the site of anatomic involvement. The aims of therapy are first to terminate the acute phase in order to achieve remission and, secondly, to maintain a quiescent phase, i.e. to prevent relapses.

There are two general possibilities for conservative treatment: namely special forms of nutrition and drugs. Since the typical feature of Crohn's disease is an unpredictable periodical course of acute attacks and quiescent phases, knowledge of the natural history of the disease has been incomplete. With respect to the natural course, therefore, this article accentuates prospective randomized controlled trials.

NUTRITION THERAPY IN CROHN'S DISEASE

Diet high in fibre, low in refined sugar

Patients with Crohn's disease seem to eat more sugar[15] and less fruit and vegetables than most people. These eating habits have been called 'pre-illness diets'[16]. Heaton *et al.*[17] therefore studied the effect of a diet with an increased fibre content and low in refined sugar in 32 patients with Crohn's disease and compared their clinical course retrospectively with that of 32 patients receiving no dietary instructions. Patients on diet had significantly fewer and shorter stays at hospital (111 *vs* 533 days) and only one *versus* five patients required surgery. Although the study received wide attention the results should be regarded with caution because only historical not randomized controls were used.

Table 3.1 Incidence (cases/100 000 per year) and prevalence (cases/100 000 inhabitants) of Crohn's disease

Authors	*Region*	*Incidence*	*Prevalence*
Kyle[2]	North-East Scotland	2.1	32.5
Binder *et al.*[3]	Copenhagen	2.7	32
Miller *et al.*[4]	Nottingham	3.6	26.5
Mayberry *et al.*[5]	Cardiff	4.8	56
Goebell *et al.*[6]	Ruhr area	4.2	36.8
Nylin *et al.*[7]	Norbotten & Västerbotten	4.9	-
Hellers[8]	Stockholm	5	54.2
Brahme *et al.*[9]	Malmö	6	75.2
Sedlack *et al.*[10]	Olmsted County	6.6	106
Nunes *et al.*[11]	Spokane	8.8	-

A first prospective controlled trial conducted by Brandes *et al.*[18] compared 10 patients subjected to a low refined carbohydrate diet with 10 controls on normal diet. The CDAI[12] fell under refined sugar restriction, whereas the clinical course under normal nutrition worsened. The problem of this study is its limitation to 20 patients.

In a very recent and most extensive report by Ritchie *et al.*[19], 190 patients were randomly allocated to a fibre-rich diet low in refined carbohydrates, and 162 to a diet unrestricted in sugar and low in fibre. This prospective multicentre double-blind trial showed no striking difference in the clinical course of the two patient groups. Taking into account the objections to the first two studies and the results of the study by Ritchie, the clinical course of Crohn's disease therefore seems to be unaffected by a reduction of refined sugar intake (Table 3.2).

Low residue diet

A prospective randomized study from Italy[20] including 70 patients with non-stenosing Crohn's disease, compared the effect of a low residue diet with an unrestricted normal Italian diet for a mean of 29 months. There was no

Table 3.2 The effect of a diet high in fibre, low in refined sugar, in Crohn's disease

Author	*No. of patients*	*Diet regimen*	*Study design*	*Period (months)*	*Comment*
Heaton[17]	32 32	Diet Unrestricted	Uncontrolled Retrospective	40	Diet beneficial in clinical course
Brandes[18]	10 10	Diet Unrestricted	Controlled Prospective	18	Decrease of CDAI in diet group
Ritchie[19]	190 162	Diet unrestricted	Controlled Prospective	24	No difference in clinical course

difference with respect to symptoms, number of hospital admissions, surgery, nutritional status, complications, or postoperative recurrence. These results led the authors to recommend a balanced diet without unnecessary restrictions on patients' eating habits which could reduce their life quality. However, since traditional Italian food is rich in fruits and vegetables, with complex carbohydrates, and low in sugar anyway, these results, as the authors point out, might not be transferrable to Northern European or other unrestricted diets.

Exclusion diet

A controlled trial, published in 1985 by V.A. Jones[21], was given great publicity. The background aim of this study was to eliminate specific foods to which patients might be intolerant. Twenty patients with quiescent Crohn's disease (CDAI <150) were randomly allocated either to an unrefined carbohydrate fibre-rich diet or to be investigated for specific food intolerances. Seven out of 10 patients on the exclusion diet remained in remission for 6 months. In contrast all patients on unrefined carbohydrate, fibre-rich diet had a relapse. Moreover, in an uncontrolled manner, 51 out of 77 patients solely on the exclusion diet remained well, the longest for 51 months, with a relapse rate of less than 10% per year. The most frequent offending foods were wheat and dairy products. The authors concluded that the exclusion diet might be an effective long-term therapeutic strategy for Crohn's disease. The study has been questioned because of the small number of patients included in the controlled trial. Another criticism was that the groups were not strictly comparable with respect to drug pretreatment and anatomic involvement of disease. Clearly, more controlled studies are necessary to substantiate these results.

Total parenteral nutrition and formula diet

Weight loss is a common feature in Crohn's disease – related to 70% of patients with an acute attack[22]. Since malnutrition is associated with increased morbidity, nutritional support, given either parenterally or enterally has been shown to be beneficial. Total parenteral nutrition (TPN) and formula diet (FD), which is absorbed in the jejunum, lead to 'bowel rest' of the damaged intestine, provided that the upper parts of the gastrointestinal tract proximal to the terminal ileum are not involved. It is believed that inflamed intestines heal better without mechanical, secretory or antigenetic exposure. Although improvements in nutritional status are well documented, the additional effect of 'bowel rest' therapy upon inflammation remains obscure.

FD, and especially TPN, are widely used as an adjunct when conventional medical therapy has failed. There are many retrospective and uncontrolled prospective studies demonstrating that nutritional support is beneficial to malnourished patients in Crohn's disease. The reported remission rates during hospital stay vary between 40 and 100% under FD[23–27] and between 28 and 100% under TPN[28–33]. It is extremely difficult to evaluate these reports since they were uncontrolled and patients often received medication such as corticosteroids or salicyl-azo-sulphapyridine (SASP).

Only a few prospective, controlled and randomized trials are reported in the literature concerning TPN in Crohn's disease. The first was conducted by Dickinson *et al.*[34]. Patients with chronic inflammatory bowel disease were subjected either to conventional therapy alone or in combination with TPN. Most of the patients had ulcerative colitis and only nine Crohn's disease – these were unequally allocated to the control (three patients) and to the TPN group (six patients). All controls yet only four in the TPN group settled. Because of the small number of patients investigated and the unequalled distribution, no conclusions can be drawn.

The second controlled trial was published by Greenberg in abstract form[35]. Three groups of patients with Crohn's disease were subjected either to TPN (17 patients), elementary diet (19 patients), or partial parenteral nutrition combined with oral nutrition. Medical treatment was continued. All three groups reached similar remission rates exhibiting no statistical difference. Thus it appears that bowel rest *per se* has no effect on the disease.

In another controlled trial[36], the influence of either TPN or oral diet on clinical course in 47 patients with severe colitis was studied. Since there were only a few patients with Crohn's disease, clinical outcome was inconclusive.

The role of formula diets in the treatment of Crohn's disease has been studied in four controlled trials. O'Morain *et al.*[37] randomized 21 patients with acute Crohn's disease to receive 0.75 mg kg^{-1} per day prednisolone or an elemental diet for 12 weeks. Both groups showed similar improvements. The authors concluded that elemental diet offers a therapeutically effective non-toxic alternative to drugs and surgery. Saverymuttu *et al.*[38] investigated 37 patients with 'moderately' active Crohn's disease and randomized them either to prednisolone 0.5 mg kg^{-1} per day plus normal diet or an elemental diet plus oral non-absorbable antibiotics (framycetin, colistin, nystatin) for a period of 10 days. Both groups improved clinically and no statistical difference was found in CDAI, ESR or fecal granulocyte excretion. It was concluded that a decrease in intraluminal, potentially allergenic food molecules and bacteria offers an alternative approach to management of Crohn's disease.

In another study by Sanderson[39], 15 children with small bowel active Crohn's disease were randomized either to elemental diet (eight children) or steroid therapy (seven children, initially treated with adrenocorticotrophic hormone 2 IU kg^{-1} per day for 5 days, followed by prednisolone 2 mg kg^{-1} per day for 30 days), combined with sulphasalazine 50 mg kg^{-1} per day. The elemental diet was just as effective as the high-dose, combined steroid and sulphasalazine therapy.

In another randomized multicenter trial (European Cooperative Crohn's Disease Study III)[40], 95 patients were allocated either to liquid defined formula diet or to drug combination therapy consisting of 6-methyl-prednisolone and sulphasalazine. After 6 weeks, 41% in the nutrition group but 73% in the drug group were in remission ($p<0.05$). However because of unpalatibility of the diet 21 in the nutrition group dropped out. Decrease in the CDAI of those patients who finished the study revealed no statistical difference between diet and drug treatment. Further analysis showed that patients with colonic involvement had a greater benefit from drug therapy.

The most extensive report was that of Lochs *et al.*[41] published in abstract form as a result of the European Cooperative Crohn's Disease Study IV: 107 patients with active Crohn's disease (CDAI >150) were investigated. 55 were assigned to a low molecular weight (oligopeptide) diet by a duodenal tube, compared with 52 patients on 6-methylprednisolone and sulphasalazine. In the diet group, 29 patients and, in the drug group, 41 patients achieved remission in median remission times of 30.7 and 8.2 days, respectively. Subgroups designated as patients with severe (CDAI >300) and less severe (CDAI <300) disease and patients with different anatomic involvement (terminal ileum, ileocolic, colic) showed no difference with respect to the therapeutic regimes. From these results it was concluded that while an enteral low molecular weight diet is effective, it is less so than combination therapy with 6-methylprednisolone and sulphasalazine (Table 3.3).

Table 3.3 Formula diets (FD) in the treatment of active Crohn's disease: prospective, randomized, controlled trials

Authors	*No. of Patients*	*Treatment*	*Duration of therapy (days)*	*Response (%)*
O'Morain *et al.*[37]	11	FD	28	80
	10	Pred	28	80
Saverymuttu *et al.*[38]	16	FD + Antib	10	94
	16	Pred	10	94
Sanderson *et al.*[39]	8	FD	42	87.5 [a]
	7	ACTH/Pred + SASP	42	85
Malchow *et al.*[40]	51	FD	42 [b]	41
	44	6-MP/SASP	42	73
Lochs *et al.*[41]	55	FD	42	53
	52	Pred + SASP	42	79

Abbreviations: Pred = prednisolone; SASP = sulphasalazine; 6-MP = 6-methylprednisolone; Antib = Antibiotics; ACTH = adrenocorticotrophic hormone
[a] At least 87.5%, one child who left the trial was regarded as a non-responder
[b] Only 31 patients completed the trial

The present investigations suggest that formula diet is an effective treatment for Crohn's disease and may offer a non-toxic alternative for all patients who respond primarily to this mode of therapy.

DRUG THERAPY IN CROHN'S DISEASE

In treating acute attacks, the drugs that have been shown to be beneficial, by controlled trials, include steroids, sulphasalazine and metronidazol. The benefit of the recently introduced drug 5-aminosalicylic acid (5-ASA) is not established in Crohn's disease. Levamisol has definitely been shown to be ineffective. Only anecdotal and uncontrolled reports exist about the efficacy of 7S-immunoglobulin and cyclosporin. Likewise, reports of treatment with tuberculostatics are completely preliminary.

To date, no available drug treatment modalities have been shown incontrovertibly successfully to prevent flare-ups.

Corticosteroids

The most important studies, with the largest number of patients, are the Crohn's disease trials of North America (NCCDS)[42] and Western Europe (ECCDS)[43]: they unequivocally demonstrated the efficacy of corticosteroids in *acute attacks of Crohn's disease*.

In the NCCDS, 569 patients were included in a multicentre, randomized, placebo-controlled trial. Prednisone given in a dose of 0.5–0.75 mg (kg b.wt.)$^{-1}$ induced remission (CDAI <150) more rapidly and more effectively than placebo did. Neither SASP nor azathioprine were as effective as prednisone.

In the ECCDS, a similar design was applied to 452 patients: 6-methylprednisolone, initially given at a dose of 48 mg, was the most effective drug compared with placebo or SASP.

Eight of the study centres participating in the NCCDS conducted a trial to answer the question as to whether the combination of prednisone, 0.5–0.75 mg (kg b.wt.)$^{-1}$, and SASP, 1 g (15 kg b.wt.)$^{-1}$, is superior to prednisone alone in acute Crohn's disease (TAS Study): 89 patients entered into a double-blind, randomized, multicentre trial. Patients taking both prednisone and SASP, 1 g (15 kg b.wt.)$^{-1}$, exhibited a poorer response than did patients taking prednisone and placebo[44]. The latter combination achieved quiescence and a lasting quiescent state significantly sooner than did the combination prednisone/SASP. Likewise the ECCDS revealed no benefit when using 6-methylprednisolone in combination with 3 g SASP compared to 6-methylprednisolone alone (Figure 3.1). However, it was also stated by the authors that the combination therapy may be advantageous in patients with colonic involvement or in patients previously untreated.

For patients in *quiescent disease*, none of the available studies could demonstrate with statistical significance that corticosteroids helped to sustain the quiescent state. Prednisone, 7.5 mg daily, failed to prevent recurrent disease after resection in patients followed for up to three years[45]. Likewise neither prednisone, 0.25 mg (kg b.wt.)$^{-1}$, in the NCCDS[42] nor 6-methylprednisolone, 8 mg per day, in the ECCDS[43] could maintain remission. In all the studies referred to above, relapses occurred in 40–60% of patients within 2 years regardless of whether they were under corticosteroids or placebo

(Table 3.4). Nevertheless, it should be mentioned that in the European study a subgroup of patients with active disease, treated with 6-methylprednisolone at entry, might have gained benefit from low-dose 6-methylprednisolone (8 mg per day) in long-term management of the disease.

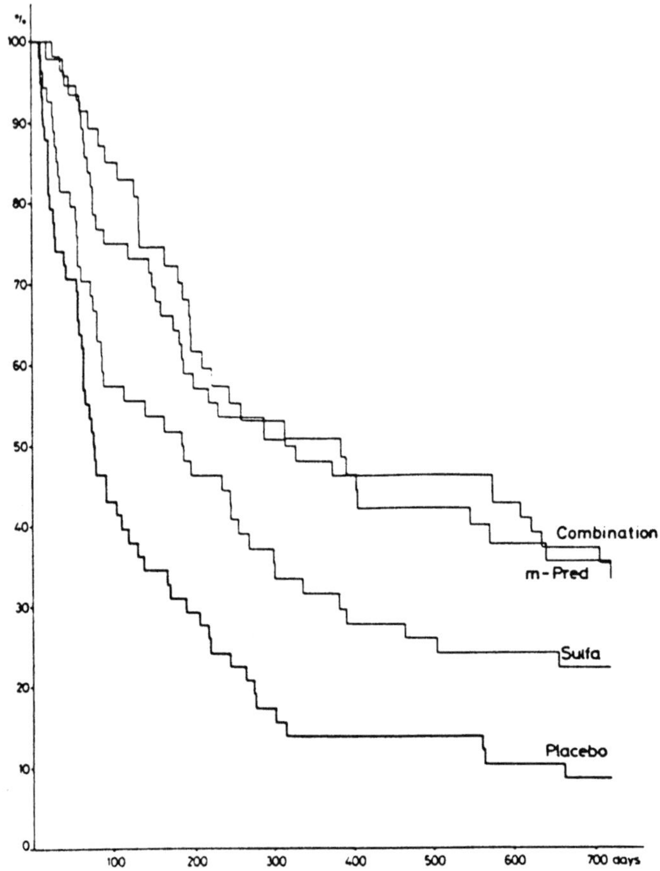

Figure 3.1 The influence of 6-methylprednisolone alone or in combination with SASP on active disease (CDAI >150)[43]. Life table analysis based on 'failure and relapse': (1) m-Pred and combination *vs* placebo: highly significant ($p<0.001$); (2) Sulfa *vs* placebo: weakly significant ($p<0.05$); other statistical methods without significant difference

Combined therapy of corticosteroids and SASP did not show any benefit in quiescent disease. In an early Scandinavian study by Bergman and Krause[46], 84 patients operated on by radical resection of the inflamed bowel were randomly divided into two groups: one group received 3 g SASP for an initial period of 16 weeks, then 1.5 g for a second period of 17 weeks.

Concomitantly, 15 mg prednisolone were administered for two weeks and 10 mg for 14 weeks, respectively, corresponding to the first period. For the second period, 5 mg were prescribed for 17 weeks. The other group received placebos. There was no statistically significant difference in the number of recurrences in the two groups of patients. The same impression was given by the TAS Study[44] and the ECCDS[43].

Table 3.4 Corticosteroids in controlled trials for maintaining remission

Authors	*No. of patients*	*Drug regimen*	*Dose (daily)*	*Observation period (months)*	*Prevention of relapse*
Summers *et al.*[42]	61	Prednisone	0.25 mg kg^{-1}	24	n.s.d.
	101	Placebo	–		
Malchow *et al.*[43]	66	6-Methylprednisolone	8.0 mg	24	n.s.d.
	52	Placebo	–		
Smith *et al.*[45]	33	Prednisone	7.5 mg	36	n.s.d.
	26	Placebo	–		

n.s.d. = no statistical difference

Salicyl-azo-sulphapyridine

The first controlled study of salicyl-azo-sulphapyridine (SASP) was a small double-blind trial of crossover design with a short treatment period of 4 weeks. It showed symptomatic improvement from SASP (3 g per day) among 17 patients with *active Crohn's disease* without previous surgery but was not advantageous for 14 patients who had developed relapse after resection[47].

In another controlled double-blind study, van Hees and coworkers[48] could demonstrate that SASP, given in a dose between 4 and 6 g per day in 13 patients, was significantly superior to placebo in 13 patients. This was independent of anatomic involvement.

The American Crohn's Disease Study demonstrated a beneficial effect of high doses of SASP, 0.1 g $(kg\ b.wt.)^{-1}$, in active disease[42], whereas lower doses of 3 g daily, employed in the European study did not exhibit a clear-cut effect[43]. In both studies, the benefit of SASP was predominantly limited to patients with Crohn's colitis.

A series of trials have failed to show that SASP maintains *quiescent disease* and reduced relapse rates[42,43,49–51].

Azathioprine and 6-mercaptopurine

The influence of azathioprine (AZA) on *acute Crohn's disease* was primarily investigated in two small double-blind crossover trials. The first study comprised 15 patients randomly allocated to either azathioprine (4 mg kg^{-1}) or placebo for 2 months with crossover to the other regime for another 2 months[52].

In the second study, 27 patients were randomized to AZA (3 mg kg^{-1}) or placebo for 4 months, followed by a 4-month period with the treatment reversed[53]. Efficacy of AZA in acute attacks could not be demonstrated in either study.

Likewise, in the NCCDS with the largest number of patients, no difference in outcome could be detected between AZA treatment (2.5 mg kg^{-1}) and the control group[42].

In *quiescent disease*, 1 mg (kg b.wt.)$^{-1}$ prescribed in the NCCDS failed to prevent relapses compared with placebo[42]. Several trials have been performed with higher doses of AZA for maintainance of quiescent Crohn's disease. A small trial, lasting 1 year was published in abstract form by Watson[54]: 11 patients were allocated either to take 50 mg AZA or placebo in a crossover design. Although the patients in the drug group felt better, no statistical difference assessed by objective parameters could be demonstrated.

Rosenberg[55] studied 20 patients for 26 weeks who took at least 10 mg prednisone prior to entering the study. They were randomized either to AZA, 2 mg (kg b.wt.)$^{-1}$, or to placebo. The average reduction in steroid dosage in the AZA group was 15.5 mg per day, in the placebo group 6.1 mg per day, demonstrating a slight but statistically significant steroid-sparing effect with AZA. In two other controlled studies[56,57], 2 mg (kg b.wt.)$^{-1}$ AZA appeared to maintain remission induced by corticosteroids. In the latter, efficacy could be demonstrated by withdrawal. Before entering the study, patients took 2 mg kg^{-1} AZA for at least 6 months. In one group this regime was continued, while the other group received placebo. The cumulative probability of relapse was 5% in the AZA group and 41% in the withdrawal group after 1 year of treatment (Table 3.5).

In an open and uncontrolled study from Sweden[58] the clinical effects of long-term immunosuppressive therapy (mean>4 years) in 42 patients with severe Crohn's disease and extensive colonic involvement were investigated; 13 patients had undergone 25 operations before treatment. At the beginning of therapy, radical surgery was not possible for 30 patients due to a currently widespread disease, the other 12 patients refused surgery and preferred a trial with medical therapy. The mean initial dose was 100 mg per day of AZA in men and 75 mg per day in women. Five patients initially took 100–150 mg daily of 6-mercaptopurine (6-MP). In four patients, AZA was changed to cyclophosphamide because of side effects. Prednisolone was given concomitantly with rapid tapering to maintenance therapy of 6.8 mg on alternate days (17 patients) or discontinuance (25 patients) within 2–3 months. The general condition improved in 37 out of 42 patients on AZA. Occurrence of complications (5/42) and operative procedures (6/42) was significantly decreased during immunosuppressive treatment, compared with the pre-treatment period (33/42 and 25/42). In 10 patients, withdrawal of all drugs was possible with an average remission period of 40 months. This uncontrolled study demonstrates the possibility of long-term immunosuppressive therapy with beneficial effects in severe and extensive Crohn's disease.

Table 3.5 Controlled trials with azathioprine (AZA) in quiescent Crohn's disease

Authors	*No. of patients*	*Drug regimen*	*Dose (per day)*	*Observation period (months)*	*Patients relapsed*
Watson & Bukowsky[54]	10	AZA/placebo crossover	50 mg	12	n.d.
Rosenberg *et al.*[55]	10	AZA	2 mg kg^{-1}	6.5	2
	10	Placebo	–	6.5	5
Willoughby *et al.*[56]	11	AZA	2 mg kg^{-1}	6	1
	11	Placebo	–	6	8
O'Donoghue *et al.*[57]	24	AZA	2 mg kg^{-1}	12	5%[a]
	27	Placebo	–	12	41%[a]
Summers *et al.*[42]	54	AZA	1 mg kg^{-1}	24	n.s.d.
	101	Placebo	–	24	

n.d. = no difference in clinical score ('better', 'same', 'worse'); n.s.d. = no statistical difference between AZA and placebo.
[a] Cumulative probability of relapse

The active metabolite of AZA, 6-mercaptopurine (6-MP), was investigated in a 2-year, randomized, double-blind partly crossover study compared with placebo in 72 chronically ill patients, in whom therapy with SASP and steroids had failed, the latter having been used many times and for long periods[59]. In most cases, active disease had once again been brought into remission with high steroid therapy. The mean initial dose of 6-MP was 1.5 mg (kg b.wt.)$^{-1}$. Abrupt cessation of cortisone was avoided. The mean time required for a response was 3.1 months. The crossover data demonstrated a 67% beneficial response during treatment with 6-MP as compared with an 8% response during placebo. The non-crossover data confirmed the superiority of 6-MP (79 *vs* 29%). Steroids could be discontinued or reduced in 75% of the 6-MP group *vs* 36% in the placebo group. Maintenance of clinical improvement was seen in 64 *vs* 15% for those on 6-MP and on placebo, respectively. Moreover, the study revealed a favourable effect of 6-MP upon the fistulae, which were closed in 31% of patients compared with 6% under placebo. With special respect to fistula healing, a subsequent study was performed partly including patients of the above study: 34 patients were treated with 6-MP for a minimum period of 6 months. Fistulae of 13 patients closed completely (39%) or improved in another nine patients (26%)[60].

Summarizing the results of the above AZA (6-MP) trials, there is no effect in acute disease and conflicting results of quiescent disease, ranging from benefit in the majority of studies to no advantage in two studies. The beneficial effect of the drug may become apparent over weeks or months rather than days at a dosage of 2 mg (kg b.wt.)$^{-1}$. In view of its potential toxicity[61], AZA should be used with reservation. Treatment is justified if all attempted conventional therapy fails and seems to be advantageous in severe Crohn's disease with extensive colonic involvement, especially in preoperated patients and patients not responding to conventional therapy. In addition, since 6-MP has been shown to be effective in treating fistulae, therapy may be tried prior to surgery.

Metronidazole

In the Swedish co-operative Crohn's disease study the effect of metronidazole (0.8 g daily) was compared with SASP (3 g daily) in patients with *active disease* (CDAI >150) in a double-blind, crossover design[62].

In the first 4 months of drug treatment, no statistical difference between the two drugs could be detected. However, in SASP non-responders of the first treatment period, metronidazole gave a significantly better response after crossover. The authors recommend switching the drug regimen to metronidazole when SASP fails. Nevertheless, because of potentially severe side effects, metronidazole should only be used as a reserve drug.

Metronidazole has been recommended for treating fistula. In a retrospective study, 18 patients with perineal Crohn's disease (predominantly fistulae) were treated with metronidazole, 20 mg kg^{-1} per day, for at least 2 months: 10 exhibited complete healing, five showed improvement[63]. A prospective trial from Germany underlined the beneficial effect of metronidazole in treating fistulae: 40% of 24 fistulae closed completely, 20%

improved by a decrease in secretion[64].

No data are available concerning a potential role of metronidazole in *quiescent disease* to prevent relapses.

5-Aminosalicylic acid

Up to now only a few studies exist on the efficacy of 5-aminosalicylic acid (5-ASA) in Crohn's disease. Enterocoated sustained-release 5-ASA tablets were employed to deliver effective topical concentrations to both the small intestine and colon[65]. The first open trial in patients with *active Crohn's disease* was reported by Rasmussen[66] who gave 1.5 g enterocoated 5-ASA to eight patients with ileitis and 10 patients with ileocolitis. The CDAI decreased significantly from a median of 226 to 99 points. The clinical course was estimated as having improved in 13 patients (72%), staying unchanged in two (11%) and becoming aggravated in three patients (17%). This study led to three further prospectively controlled trials.

Maier[67] compared the therapeutic efficacy of 5-ASA (1.5 g daily) with that of SASP (3 g daily) in 60 patients with chronic inflammatory bowel disease, 30 patients had Crohn's disease. Disease activity fell significantly within 8 weeks in 87% of the 5-ASA group and 80% of the SASP group, with no side effects in the 5-ASA group. A concomitant drug treatment with corticosteroids was undertaken in 13 patients. No data were given about the anatomic site of disease.

In a double-blind, placebo-controlled trial, Saverymuttu[68] treated 12 patients with mild to moderate Crohn's colitis with 5-ASA, 1.5 g per day, or placebo for a short period of 10 days. No significant changes (as assessed by the CDAI) were observed but a 5% decrease of ^{111}In-labelled fecal granulocytes in the 5-ASA group was observed.

In a 16-week, double-blind, placebo-controlled, multicentre study from Denmark[69], 30 patients received 5-ASA given in a dose of 1.5 g per day, 37 patients received placebo. Crohn's disease in mild or moderate form was exclusively confined to the terminal ileum. In the 5-ASA group, 40% of the patients improved *versus* 30% of the placebo-treated group. No statistically significant differences in outcome could be demonstrated.

In a German multicentre, double-blinded prospective study[70], 28 patients took 5-ASA, 2 g per day, and 27 patients were treated 'conventionally' with 6-methylprednisolone with an initial dose of 48 mg, stepwise reduced afterwards. All patients had active disease (CDAI >150). In 22 patients of the 5-ASA group (78.6%), therapy had to be interrupted because of deterioration. In the methylprednisolone group, lack of efficacy was observed in only 37%. Although preliminary, the data clearly demonstrate the superiority of methylprednisolone in active Crohn's disease[70]. Thus, on the basis of present results, 5-ASA cannot be recommended as monotherapy in *active Crohn's disease* (Table 3.6).

For *quiescent disease* no data are available to answer the question as to whether 5-ASA is suitable for maintenance of remission or not.

Table 3.6 Controlled trials with 5-aminosalicylic acid (5-ASA) in active Crohn's disease

Authors	*No. of Patients*	*Drug*	*Dose (daily)*	*Treatment period*	*Comment*
Maier *et al.*[67]	15 [a]	5-ASA	1.5 g	8 weeks	CDAI-index from 308 to 111; $p<0.0001$
	15 [b]	SASP	3.0 g	8 weeks	310 to 162; $p<0.0001$
Saverymuttu *et al.*[68]	6	5-ASA	1.5 g	10 days	No change in CDAI index, 5% decrease of ^{111}In-labelled fecal granulocytes in 5-ASA group
	6	Placebo	–	10 days	
Rassmussen *et al.*[69]	30	5-ASA	1.5 g	16 weeks	40% in 5-ASA group and 30% in placebo group improved; no statistical difference
	37	Placebo	–	16 weeks	
Jens *et al.*[70]	28	5-ASA	2.0 g	24 weeks	78.6% deterioration in 5-ASA group, 37% in 6-Met-P-group
	27	6-Met-P	48 mg [c]	24 weeks	

[a] six patients ([b] seven patients) with concomitant corticoid medication
[c] initial dosage with weekly tapering
6-Met-P = 6-methylprednisolone

Other drugs

Levamisole

Levamisole is a synthetic anti-helminthic drug with cellular immuno-stimulating potency. After an encouraging uncontrolled study[71], an early[72] and a recently published controlled trial[73] did not show any obvious efficacy of levamisole in *active Crohn's disease.*

Likewise, a recent multicentre prospective, double-blind controlled trial from France, including 155 patients with *quiescent Crohn's disease* offered no significant difference between placebo and levamisole-treated patient groups with respect to occurrence of flare-up[74].

7S-Immunoglobulin

7S-Immunoglobulin was given intravenously to three patients with active Crohn's disease, of whom two were refractory to conventional therapy with steroids and SASP. Their condition improved within a few days – as assessed by CDAI and special laboratory indices (antitrypsin, orosomucoid)[75]. A controlled trial is in progress.

Cyclosporin A

Since immunological mechanisms in the aetiology of Crohn's disease are being discussed, cyclosporin may be beneficial by modulating the cellular immune response. No controlled trials are available up to now. Experience with cyclosporin A is limited to anecdotal reports[76] and a few open trials predominantly published in abstract form.

In a Canadian open study, 10 patients with acute Crohn's disease (CDA>150), reported an initial oral dose of 10 mg $(kg\ b.wt.)^{-1}$ of cyclosporin A serum trough level between 100 and 200 ng ml^{-1} for 16 weeks. Improvement occured early within 4 weeks for all patients, yet three out of 10 relapsed. Within 4 weeks of stopping cyclosporin A, four of the remaining seven patients relapsed[77]. In another study, eight of 11 patients improved within 3 months. Follow-up data in five patients 0–3 months after tapering off revealed that only three had improved still further, and two patients had worsened[78].

Likewise, in a small study from the UK, eight patients unresponsive to combinations of prednisolone, azathioprine, and SASP received cyclosporin A for 6 weeks, with the dosage adjusted to blood levels. Seven of eight patients responded to cyclosporin with symptomatic improvement, weight gain and return of C-reactive protein to normal. However, after cessation of cyclosporin severe relapse occurred in three patients[79].

Thus, at the present time, the role of cyclosporin A in the treatment of Crohn's disease still remains to be clearly defined. Controlled trials are expected to substantiate potential benefit.

Tuberculostatics

There are several uncontrolled studies in abstract form which deal with tuberculostatics in the therapy of Crohn's disease. They are based upon the fact that atypical mycobacteria were isolated from the tissue of patients with Crohn's disease[80,81,82].

Rutgeerts[83] employed for six months a combination therapy with rifabutin (5 mg kg^{-1}) and ethambutol (15 mg kg^{-1}), which failed to affect activity in seven patients.

In contrast, another uncontrolled study consisting of six patients with 'severe refractory Crohn's disease or repetitive resistant fistulization and abscess formation' who improved during therapy with streptomycin (1 g for 5 days a week over 2–4 months) and rifabutin (0.3 g daily) in CDAI, could be withdrawn from steroids and showed healing of fistulae[84].

Quadruple anti-mycobacterial therapy (rifampicin, isoniazid, ethambutol and pyrazinamide) was given to 17 patients with active Crohn's disease for 6 months: 12 patients improved with a significant fall of CDAI[85].

The present preliminary data warrant controlled trials in order to assess the role of tuberculostatics in Crohn's disease.

SUMMARY

Summarizing the present studies with respect to conservative therapy in Crohn's disease, the question is: 'How should a patient be treated with Crohn's disease today?'

If a patient is admitted for *active disease*, the drug of choice is clearly prednisolone (prednisone or 6-methylprednisolone), initially given at a dose of 60 mg daily (or equivalent), particularly when disease is confined to the terminal ileum. A combination with SASP might be advantageous in patients with ileocolitis. Crohn's colitis can be treated with SASP alone yet at a high dose. SASP can probably be replaced by 5-ASA, because the latter is the effective part of SASP with much fewer side effects. For patients who refuse or do not tolerate steroid therapy because of severe side effects, a low molecular weight diet can be tried as an alternative.

Patients with poor nutritional status who are not capable of oral intake of sufficient calories, with possible electrolyte imbalance because of profuse diarrhoea or i.e. with subileus, should contemporaneously be nourished by adjuvant total parenteral nutrition.

In the case of fistulae, treatment with 6-MP, 1.5 mg kg^{-1} per day, or metronidazole, 0.8–1 g per day, is appropriate for at least 2–3 months prior to surgery.

In *quiescent disease* no established therapeutic regimen is available to date. After having induced remission, a low dose of prednisolone ($<$7.5 mg daily) might have a beneficial influence on the clinical course yet strong evidence for efficacy is lacking. AZA, 2 mg kg^{-1} (6-MP, 1.5 mg daily) may be suitable for long-term treatment in chronically ill patients with extensive disease, where other long-term conventional treatment has failed.

REFERENCES

1. Crohn, B.B., Ginzburg, L. and Oppenheimer, G.D. (1932). Regional ileitis. A pathological and clinical entity. *J. Am. Med. Assoc.*, **99**, 1323–9
2. Kyle, J. (1971). An epidemiological study of Crohn's disease in North East Scotland. *Gastroenterology*, **61**, 826–33
3. Binder, V., Both, H., Hansen, P.K. *et al.* (1982). Incidence and prevalence of ulcerative colitis and Crohn's disease in the County of Kopenhagen 1962–1978. *Gastroenterology*, **83**, 563–8
4. Miller, D.S., Keighly, A.C. and Langman, M.J.S. (1974). Changing patterns in epidemiology of Crohn's disease. *Lancet*, **2**, 691–3
5. Mayberry, J.F., Rhodes, J. and Hughes, L.E. (1979). Incidence of Crohn's disease in Cardiff between 1934 and 1977. *Gut*, **20**, 602–8
6. Goebell, H., Dirks, E. and Förster, S. (1987). Prospective analysis of the frequency of chronic inflammatory bowel disease in an urban population (Ruhr Area). In: Goebell, H., Peskar, B.M. and Malchow, H. (eds.) *Inflammatory Bowel Disease*, pp. 241–2. (Lancaster: MTP Press)
7. Nylin, H. and Danielsson, A. (1986). Incidence of Crohn's disease in a defined population in Northern Sweden, 1974–1981. *Scand. J. Gastroenterol.*, **21**, 1185–92
8. Heller, G. (1979). Crohn's disease in Stockholm County 1955–1974. A study of epidemiology, results of surgical treatment and long-term prognosis. *Act. Chir. Scand.*, **490** (suppl.), 1–84
9. Brahme, F., Lindstrom, C. and Wenckert, A. (1975). Crohn's disease in a defined population. An epidemiological study of incidence, prevalence, mortality and secular trends in the city of Malmö, Sweden. *Gastroenterology*, **69**, 342–51
10. Sedleck, R.E., Whisnant, J., Elveback, L.R. *et al.* (1980). Incidence of Crohn's disease in Olmsted County, Minnesota, 1935–1975. *Am. J. Epidemiol.*, **112**, 759–63
11. Nunes, G.C. and Ahlquist, R.E. (1983). Increasing incidence of Crohn's disease. *Am. J. Surg.*, **145**, 578–81
12. Best, W.R., Becktel, J.M., Singleton, J.W. and Kern, F. (1976). Development of a Crohn's Disease Activity Index. *Gastroenterology*, **70**, 439–44
13. Van Hees, P.A.M., Van Elteren, P.H., van Lier, H.J.J. and van Tongeren, J.H.M. (1980). An index of inflammatory activity in patients with Crohn's disease. *Gut*, **21**, 279–86
14. Harvey, R.F. and Bradshaw, J.M. (1980). A simple index of Crohn's disease activity. *Lancet*, **1**, 514–5
15. Martini, G.A. and Brandes, J.W. (1976). Increased consumption of refined carbohydrates in patients with Crohn's disease. *Klin. Wschr.*, **54**, 367–71
16. Thornton, J.R., Emmet, P.M. and Heaton, K.W. (1979). Diet and Crohn's disease: characteristics of the pre-illness diet. *Br. Med. J.*, **2**, 762–4
17. Heaton, K.W., Thornton, J.R. and Emmet, P.M. (1979). Treatment of Crohn's disease with an unrefined-carbohydrate fibre-rich diet. *Br. Med. J.*, **2**, 764–6
18. Brandes, J.W. and Lorenz-Meyer, H. (1981). Zuckerfreie Diät: Eine neue Perspektive zur Behandlung des Morbus Crohn? *Z. Gastroenterol.*, **19**, 1–12
19. Ritchie, J.K., Wadsworth, J., Lennard-Jones, J.E. and Rogers, E. (1987). Controlled multicentre therapeutic trial of an unrefined carbohydrate, fibre-rich diet in Crohn's disease. *Br. Med. J.*, **295**, 517–20
20. Levenstein, S., Prantera, C., Luzi, C. and D'Ubaldi, A. (1985). Low residue or normal diet in Crohn's disease: a prospective controlled study in Italian patients. *Gut*, **26**, 989–93
21. Jones, V.A., Workman, E., Freeman, A.H., Dickinson, R.J., Wilson, A.J. and Hunter, J.O. (1985). Crohn's disease: Maintenance of remission by diet. *Lancet*, **2**, 177–80
22. Driscoll, R.H. and Rosenberg, I.H. (1978). Total parenteral nutrition in inflammatory bowel disease. *Med. Clin. North Am.*, **62**, 185–201
23. Voitk, A.J., Echave, V., Feller, J.H. *et al.* (1973). Experience with elemental diet in the treatment of inflammatory bowel disease. *Arch. Surg.*, **107**, 329–33

24. Morin, C.L., Roulet, M., Weber, A., Roy, C.C. *et al.* (1979). Nasogastric infusion of elemental diet (ED) as a primary therapy in Crohn's disease. *Pediatr. Res.*, **13**, 405 (abstract)
25. Hylander, E. and Jarnum, S. (1980). Klinische Erfahrungen mit Elementardiäten bei gastro-intestinalen Erkrankungen. *Akt. Ernährungsmed*, **5**, 105–7
26. Lochs, H.M., Egger-Schödl, M., Schuh, R. *et al.* (1984). Is tube feeding with elemental diets a primary therapy of Crohn's disease? *Klin. Wschr.*, **62**, 821–5
27. Teahon, K., Bjarnason, I. and Levi, A.J. (1988). Elemental diet in the management of Crohn's disease. A 10-year review. *Gastroenterology*, **94**, A457
28. Bos, L.P. and Weterman, I.T. (1980). Total parenteral nutrition in Crohn's disease. *World J. Surg.*, **4**, 163–6
29. Reilly, J., Ryan, J.A., Strole, W. and Fischer, J.E. (1976). Hyperalimentation in inflammatory bowel disease. *Am. J. Surg.*, **131**, 192–200
30. Elson, C.O., Layden, T.J., Nemchausky, B.A. (1980). An evaluation of total parenteral nutrition in the management of inflammatory bowel disease. *Dig. Dis. Sci.*, **25**, 42–8
31. Ostro, M.J., Greenberg, J.R. and Jeejeebhoy, K.N. (1985). Total parenteral nutrition and complete bowel rest in the management of Crohn's disease. *J. Parent. Ent. Nutr.*, **9**, 280–7
32. Müller, J.M., Keller, H.W., Erasmi, H. and Pichlmaier, H. (1983). Total parenteral nutrition as the sole therapy in Crohn's disease – a prospective study. *Br. J. Surg.*, **70**, 40–3
33. Shiloni, E. and Freund, H.R. (1983). Total parenteral nutrition in Crohn's disease. Is it a primary or supportive mode of therapy? *Dis. Colon Rectum*, **26**, 275–8
34. Dickinson, R.J., Ashton, M.G., Axon, A.T.R. *et al.* (1980). Controlled trial of intravenous hyperalimentation and total bowel rest as an adjunct to the routine therapy of acute colitis. *Gastroenterology*, **79**, 1199–204
35. Greenberg, G.R., Fleming, C.R., Jeejeebhoy, K.N. *et al.* (1985). Controlled trial of bowel rest and nutritional support in the management of Crohn's disease. *Gastroenterology*, **88**, 1405 (abstract)
36. McIntyre, P.B., Powell-Tuck, J., Wood, S.R. *et al.* (1986). Controlled trial of bowel rest in the treatment of severe acute colitis. *Gut*, **27**, 481–5
37. O'Morain, C., Segal, A.W. and Levi, A.J. (1984). Elemental diet as a primary treatment of acute Crohn's disease: a controlled trial. *Br. Med. J.*, **288**, 1859–62
38. Saverymuttu, S., Hodgson, H.J.F. and Chadwick, V.S. (1985). Controlled trial comparing prednisolone with an elemental diet plus non-absorbable antibiotics in active Crohn's disease. *Gut*, **26**, 994–8
39. Sanderson, I.R., Udeen, S., Davies, P.S.W. *et al.* (1987). Remission induced by an elemental diet in small bowel Crohn's disease. *Arch. Dis. Child.*, **61**, 123–7
40. Malchow, H., Steinhardt, H.J., Strohm, W.D. *et al.* (1985). Feasibility and effectiveness of a defined formula diet regimen in treating active Crohn's disease. *Gastroenterology*, **88**, 1487 (abstract)
41. Lochs, H., Steinhardt, H.J., Klaus-Wenz, B. *et al.* (1988). Enteral nutrition versus drug treatment for the acute phase of Crohn's disease: Results of the European Co-operative Crohn's Disease Study IV. *Gastroenterology*, **94**, A267
42. Summers, R.W., Switz, D.M., Sessions, J.T. *et al.* (1979). National Co-operative Crohn's Disease Study: results of drug treatment. *Gastroenterology*, **77**, 847–69
43. Malchow, H., Ewe, K., Brandes, J.W., Goebell, H. *et al.* (1984). European Cooperative Crohn's Disease Study (ECCDS): results of drug treatment. *Gastroenterology*, **86**, 249–66
44. Singleton, J.W., Summers, R.W., Kern, F. *et al.* (1979). A trial of sulfasalazine as adjunctive therapy in Crohn's disease. *Gastroenterology*, **77**, 887–97
45. Smith, R.C., Rhodes, J., Heatley, R.V. *et al.* (1978). Low dose steroids and clinical relapse in Crohn's disease: a controlled trial. *Gut*, **19**, 606–10
46. Bergman, L. and Krause, U. (1976). Postoperative treatment with corticosteroids and salazosulphapyridine (salazopyrin) after radical resection for Crohn's disease. *Scand. J. Gastroenterol.*, **11**, 651–6
47. Anthonisen, P., Barany, F., Folkenborg, O. *et al.* (1974). The clinical effect of salazosulphapyridine (salazopyrin) in Crohn's disease. *Scand. J. Gastroenterol.*, **9**, 549–54

48. Van Hees, P.A.M., van Lier, H.J.J., van Elteren, P.H., Driessen, W.M.M., van Hogezand, R.A. *et al.* (1981). Effect of sulphasalazine in patients with active Crohn's disease: a controlled double blind study. *Gut*, **22**, 404–9
49. Baron, J.H., Bennett, P.N., Lennard-Jones, J.E. *et al.* (1977). Sulphasalazine in asymptomatic Crohn's disease. A multicentre trial. *Gut*, **18**, 69–72
50. Wenckert, A., Kristensen, M., Eklund, A.E. *et al.* (1978). The long-term prophylactic effect of salazosulphapyridine (salazopyrin) in primarily resected patients with Crohn's disease. *Scand. J. Gastroenterol.*, **13**, 161–7
51. Ewe, K., Malchow, H. and Herfarth, Ch. (1985). Operative Radikalität und Rezidivprophylaxe mit Azulfidine bei Morbus Crohn: Ein prospektive multicentrische Studie. *Langenbecks Arch. Chir.*, **364**, 427–30
52. Rhodes, J., Beck, P., Bainton, D. and Campbell, H. (1971). Controlled trial of azathioprine in Crohn's disease. *Lancet*, **12**, 1273–6
53. Klein, M., Binder, H.J., Mitchel, M *et al.* (1974). Treatment of Crohn's disease with azathioprine: a controlled evaluation. *Gastroenterology*, **66**, 916–22
54. Watson, W.C. and Bukowsky, M. (1974). Azathioprine in management of Crohn's disease: a randomized crossover study. *Gastroenterology*, **66**, A142
55. Rosenberg, J.L., Levin, B., Wall, A.J. and Kirsner, J.B. (1975). A controlled trial of azathioprine in Crohn's disease. *Dig. Dis.*, **20**, 721–6
56. Willoughby, J.M.T., Beckett, J., Kumar, P.J. *et al.* (1971). Controlled trial of azathioprine in Crohn's disease. *Lancet*, **2**, 944–6
57. O'Donnoghue, D.P., Dawson, A.M., Powell-Tuck, J. *et al.* (1978). Double blind withdrawal trial of azathioprine as maintenance treatment for Crohn's disease. *Lancet*, **2**, 955–7
58. Nyman, M., Hansson, I. and Eriksson, S. (1985). Long-term immunosupressive treatment in Crohn's disease. *Scand. J. Gastroenterol.*, **20**, 1197–203
59. Present, D.H., Korelitz, B.I., Wisch, N. *et al.* (1980). Treatment of Crohn's disease with 6-mercaptopurine. *N. Engl. J. Med.*, **302**, 981–7
60. Korelitz, B.I. and Present, D.H. (1985). Favorable effect of 6-mercaptopurine on fistulae of Crohn's disease. *Dig. Dis. Sci.*, **30**, 58–64
61. Singleton, J.W., Law, D.H., Kelley, M.L. *et al.* (1979). National Co-operative Crohn's Disease Study: adverse reaction to study drugs. *Gastroenterology*, **77**, 870–82
62. Rosen, A., Ursing, B., Alm, Th., Barany, F. *et al.* (1982). A comparative study of metronidazole and sulfasalazine for active Crohn's disease: The Co-operative Crohn's Disease Study in Sweden. *Gastroenterology*, **83**, 541–9
63. Bernstein, L.H., Frank, M.S., Brandt, L.J. *et al.* (1980). Healing of perineal Crohn's disease with metronidazole. *Gastroenterology*, **79**, 357–65
64. Schneider, M.U., Laudage, G., Guggenmoos-Holzmann, I. and Riemann, J.F. (1985). Metronidazol in der Behandlung des Morbus Crohn. *Dtsch. Med. Wschr.*, **110**, 1724–30
65. Rasmussen, S.N., Bondesen, S., Hvidberg, E.F. *et al.* (1982). 5-Aminosalicylic acid in a slow release preparation: Bioavailability, plasma level and excretion in humans. *Gastroenterology*, **83**, 1062–70
66. Rasmussen, S.N., Binder, V., Maier, K. *et al.* (1983). Treatment of Crohn's disease with peroral 5-aminosalicylic acid. *Gastroenterology*, **85**, 1350–3
67. Maier, K., Frühmorgen, P., Bode, J. Ch. *et al.* (1985). Erfolgreiche Akutbehandlung chronisch-entzündlicher Darmerkrankungen mit oraler 5-Aminosalicylsäure. *Dtsch. Med. Wschr.*, **110**, 363–8
68. Saverymuttu, S.H., Gupta, S., Keshavarzian, A. *et al.* (1986). Effect of a slow release 5-aminosalicylic acid preparation on disease activity in Crohn's disease. *Digestion*, **33**, 89–91
69. Rasmussen, S.N., Lauritsen, K., Tage-Jensen, U. *et al.* (1987). 5-Aminosalicylic acid in the treatment of Crohn's disease. *Scand. J. Gastroenterol.*, **22**, 877–33
70. Jenss, H., Hartmann, F. and Schölmerich, J. (1988). Therapie des aktiven Morbus Crohn mit 5-Aminosalicylsäure oder Methylprednisolon. *Z. Gastroenterol.*, (Abstract) **24**, 473
71. Segal, A.W., Levi, A.J. and Loewi, G. (1977). Levamisole in the treatment of Crohn's disease. *Lancet*, **2**, 382–4
72. Wesdorp, E., Schellekens, P.T.A., Weening, R. *et al.* (1978). Levamisole in Crohn's disease. *Digestion*, **18**, 186–91

73. Sachar, D.B., Rubin, K.P. and Gumaste, V. (1987). Levamisole in Crohn's disease: a randomized, double-blind, placebo-controlled clinical trial. *Am. J. Gastroenterol.*, **82**, 536–9
74. Modigliani, R., Pieddeloup, C., Hecketsweiler, P. *et al.* (1983). Effet du levamisole sur la prevention des pousees evolutives de la maladie de Crohn quiescente. *Gastroenterol. Clin. Biol.*, **7**, 683–92
75. Rohr, G., Kusterer, K., Schille, M. *et al.* (1987). Treatment of Crohn's disease and ulcerative colitis with 7S-immunoglobulin. *Lancet*, **1**, 170 (letter)
76. Allison, M.C. and Pounder, R.E. (1984). Cyclosporin for Crohn's disease. *Lancet*, **1**, 902–3 (letter)
77. Peltekian, K.M., Williams, C.N., MacDonald, A.S. *et al.* (1987). Open study of cyclosporin A in Crohn's disease. *Gastroenterology*, **92**, 1571 (abstract)
78. Brynskov, J., Binder, V., Riis, P. *et al.* (1987). Clinical experience with cyclosporin (cyclosporin A) in chronically-active, therapy-resistant Crohn's disease. A pilot study. *Gastroenterology*, **92**, 1330 (abstract)
79. Allison, M.C. and Pounder, R.E. (1987). Cyclosporin for Crohn's disease. *Aliment. Pharmacol. Ther.*, **1**, 39–43
80. Chiodini, R.J., van Kruiningen, H.J., Thayer, W.R., Merkal, R.S. and Coutu, J.A. (1984). Possible role of mycobacteria in inflammatory bowel disease. I. An unclassified mycobacterium species isolated from patients with Crohn's disease. *Dig. Dis. Sci.*, **29**, 1073–9
81. McFadden J.J., Butcher, P.D., Chiodini, R. and Hermon-Taylor, J. (1987). Crohn's disease isolated mycobacteria are identical to *Mycobacterium paratuberculosis*, as determined by DNA-probes that distinguish between mycobacterial species. *J. Clin. Microbiol.*, **25**, 796–801
82. Gitnick, G. (1984). Is Crohn's disease a mycobacterial disease after all? *Dig. Dis. Sci.*, **25**, 1086–8
83. Rutgerts, P., Vantrappen, G., Van Isfeldt, K. *et al.* (1988). Rifabutin therapy in patients with recurrent Crohn's disease after ileocolonic resection. *Gastroenterology*, **94**, A391
84. Thayer, W.R., Coutu, J.A., Chiodini, R.A. *et al.* (1988). Use of rifabutin and streptomycin in the therapy of Crohn's disease. *Gastroenterology*, **94**, A458
85. Hampson, S.J., Parker, M.C., Saverymuttu, S.H. *et al.* (1988). Results of quadruple antimycobacterial chemotherapy in 17 Crohn's disease patients completing six months treatment. *Gastroenterology*, **94**, A170

4
Progress in nutritional management of patients with Crohn's disease

H. LOCHS AND A. GANGL

INTRODUCTION

As with many other diseases of the gastrointestinal tract there have been several attempts to treat patients with Crohn's disease with nutritional therapy. If one analyses these attempts one can find three different approaches:

(1) It was hypothesized that Crohn's disease is caused by special dietary habits and therefore changing of these habits should avoid or heal Crohn's disease. Consequently special diets were recommended for patients with inactive Crohn's disease.

(2) Patients with Crohn's disease clearly experience food-dependent symptoms. Therefore parenteral and enteral nutrition regimens have been used to avoid these symptoms. Different investigators observed that parenteral and enteral nutrition not only have a symptomatic effect but may also be a primary treatment in the acute phase of Crohn's disease.

(3) Crohn's disease leads in a good proportion of patients to nutritional deficiencies which may be caused by malabsorption due to high disease activity or multiple intestinal resections or by anorexia because of food-dependent symptoms. These malnourished patients have to be treated nutritionally regardless of whether the disease is active or inactive.

In this chapter we will try to give an overview of the literature on these three nutritional approaches to management of patients with Crohn's disease. In addition we shall attempt to comment briefly on how nutritional therapy should be carried out in accordance with present knowledge.

DIETARY TREATMENT OF INACTIVE CROHN'S DISEASE

Crohn's disease was first described some 50 years ago and shows a characteristic geographical and ethnic distribution. It is more common in civilized Western countries and within these countries some ethnic groups, like the Jewish population in the USA, more frequently suffer from Crohn's disease than others[1,2]. These epidemiological features led to the conclusion that eating habits might have causative effects in Crohn's disease. Consequently the eating habits of Crohn's patients were compared with the general population in several studies[3–14]. Table 4.1 summarizes the results of these studies. In some investigations it was shown that Crohn's patients ate more refined sugar or more carbohydrates even before the onset of their disease than a comparable healthy population. Furthermore, in some of these studies it has also been shown that Crohn's patients ate less fibre than normal controls. This finding, however, was not confirmed in other studies (Table 4.1).

Table 4.1 Sugar and fibre consumed by patients with Crohn's disease compared to healthy controls

Authors	*Year*	*Sugar*	*Fibre*
Martini & Brandes[4]	1976	↑↑	–
Miller *et al.*[5]	1976	↑↑	–
James[6]	1977	–	↑
Rawcliffe *et al.*[7]	1978	–	↓
Thornton *et al.*[8]	1979	↑↑	↓
Kasper & Sommer[9]	1979	↑↑	↑
Mayberry *et al.*[10]	1980	↑↑	–
Silkoff *et al.*[11]	1980	↑	–
Mayberry *et al.*[12]	1981	=/↑	=
Naujoks-Heinrich[13]	1982	↑↑	↓
Järnerot *et al.*[14]	1983	↑	–

↑ higher, ↓ lower, = equal consumption in Crohn's patients, – not investigated

Guthy *et al.*[15] correlated the frequency of Crohn's disease and *per capita* consumption of margarine over the period since the Second World War and found that these two curves correlated very well in some Western European countries. They concluded that margarine might have a causative effect on

Crohn's disease. However, they could not yet confirm their data in a prospective animal study.

These studies led to the conclusion that changing the eating habits of patients with Crohn's disease should inhibit the recurrence of the disease. Several dietary studies have therefore been performed with Crohn's patients. Brandes *et al.*[16] studied the effect of a diet low in refined carbohydrates and high in fibre, compared with an *ad libitum* diet containing significantly more refined carbohydrates, in a randomized study in patients with non-active Crohn's disease. They followed both groups of patients for 2 years and compared the activity index of the disease in both groups. No differences in disease activity could be seen between the two groups over the 2 years. However, a small number of patients on the *ad libitum* diet showed a recurrence very early in the study. The number, however, was not big enough to make a significant difference between the two groups. The conclusion of the authors was that a diet low in refined carbohydrates does not confer any advantages on patients with non-active Crohn's disease. A very similar study has recently been published in the UK[17]. In this study, also, the effect of a low carbohydrate diet on the disease activity in patients with non-active Crohn's disease was investigated. Although this study comprises 352 patients from 40 hospitals all over England, and efforts were made not only to document the amount of carbohydrates consumed but also the amount of fibre in the diets, here too no advantage could be shown for a low carbohydrate diet over the 2-year study period.

A different approach was used by Jones *et al.*[18] who investigated the effect of a so-called 'exclusion diet' in patients who had recovered from an acute phase of Crohn's disease by means of enteral nutrition. These patients were first treated with enteral nutrition only. They then received more and more different foods in a stepwise manner. Whenever they felt symptoms of Crohn's disease after the addition of one item this item was excluded from their diet. After 2–3 weeks, an individual exclusion diet was developed for each patient, which only included those food items which had been tolerated well. The number of items which produced symptoms in different patients was very big and also included things like tapwater. Compared to a control group, who ate normal diet enriched with fibre, the group of patients eating the exclusion diet had fewer recurrences over a control period of 6 months. This positive trend has now continued up to 5 years in a few patients[19]. However, only a rather small number of patients was included and the results have yet to be confirmed by anyone else.

In summary, therefore, it has to be concluded that at the moment there is no evidence that any dietary treatment delays or avoids recurrences in patients with non-active Crohn's disease.

NUTRITIONAL TREATMENT OF ACTIVE CROHN'S DISEASE

Patients with active Crohn's disease clearly show food-dependent symptoms, which often lead to anorexia[20]. This is followed by weight loss, negative nitrogen balance, malnutrition and multiple nutritional deficiencies[20]. Table 4.2 summarizes the most frequent nutritional deficiencies in patients with active Crohn's disease. In children, malnutrition due to active phases of Crohn's disease can be so severe that growth retardation may result[21]. In such patients nutritional therapy can be used as primary treatment of the acute inflammation and at the same time as treatment of malnutrition.

Table 4.2 Frequency of nutritional deficiencies in patients with Crohn's disease[20]

Deficiency	*Frequency (%)*
Weight loss	65 – 75
Hypoalbuminaemia	25 – 80
Intestinal protein loss	75
Negative nitrogen balance	69
Anaemia	60 – 80
Iron deficiency	39
Vitamin B_{12} deficiency	48
Folic acid deficiency	54
Ca^{2+} deficiency	13
Mg^{2+} deficiency	14 – 33
K^{+} deficiency	6 – 20
Vitamin A deficiency	11
Vitamin B_1 deficiency	+
Vitamin C deficiency	+
Vitamin D deficiency	75
Vitamin K deficiency	+
Zn^{2+} deficiency	+
Cu^{2+} deficiency	+
Metabolic bone disease	+

+ indicates described without frequency

In both indications, nutritional therapy has been shown to be successful. In several studies it could be shown that parenteral nutrition, as the sole treatment for the acute phase of Crohn's disease, leads to remission in a variable percentage of patients (Table 4.3). It was hypothesized that 'bowel rest' may be the mechanism by which parenteral nutrition heals the inflammation[24]. However, in most reports on parenteral nutrition in the acute phase of Crohn's disease the effect of improving the nutritional status could not be differentiated from the effect of bowel rest. We have compared two groups of patients with active Crohn's disease: one treated with parenteral nutrition as the only therapy and total bowel rest; the other group received parenteral nutrition and additional oral nutrition[28]. There was no significant difference in the number of patients achieving remission by the two treatments nor in the time needed to reach remission. Therefore we concluded that bowel rest cannot be the mechanism by which parenteral nutrition treats the active phase of Crohn's disease. A similar study has recently been published with the same results[34]. This conclusion is, furthermore, supported by much research published in the meantime showing that enteral nutrition works as well as parenteral nutrition as therapy for the acute phase of Crohn's disease (Table 4.3).

Table 4.3 Indication and therapeutic effect of nutritional therapy in the acute phase of inflammatory bowel disease

Authors	*Year*	*Therapy*	*Patients*	*(n)*	*Remission (%)*
Peters[22]	1976	EN + PN	CD	84	100
Fromm *et al.*[23]	1978	EN + PN	CD	23	100
Dickinson *et al.*[24]	1980	TPN	CD + UC	19	53
Kirschner *et al.*[25]	1981	EN + PN	CD	7	100
Meryn *et al.*[26]	1982	TPN	CD	23	100
Morin *et al.*[27]	1982	EN	CD	10	100
Lochs *et al.*[28]	1983	EN + PN	CD	20	75
Müller *et al.*[29]	1983	TPN	CD	25	80
Lochs *et al.*[30]	1984	EN + PN	CD	25	100 (small bowel) 50 (colon)
Ostro *et al.*[31]	1985	TPN	CD	100	77
Lerebours *et al.*[32]	1986	TPN	CD	20	95
Rabast *et al.*[33]	1986	EN	CD + UC	26	100
Greenberg *et al.*[34]	1988	PN	CD	17	71
		EN	CD	19	58
Lochs *et al.*[35]	1988	EN	CD	55	53

CD = Crohn's disease; UC = ulcerative colitis; EN = enteral nutrition; PN = parenteral nutrition; TPN = total parenteral nutrition

Regarding the improvement of the nutritional status of patients with active Crohn's disease, an increase in body weight and in the concentration of different plasma proteins could be demonstrated[26]. In children with growth retardation, growth could be induced by enteral nutrition[21,25]. Investigation of the influence of parenteral nutrition on leucine turnover as a parameter of protein turnover in Crohn's patients has shown that leucine oxidation was reduced by parenteral nutrition while leucine incorporation into protein was increased, indicating reduction of protein catabolism and increasing protein synthesis[36]. These changes were also accompanied by a significant increase in nitrogen balance, indicating that anabolism was enhanced by parenteral nutrition.

Although the exact mechanism by which nutritional therapy influences active Crohn's disease is not yet clear, the fact remains that parenteral nutrition and enteral nutrition have been used successfully to treat active phases of the disease. Improvement of the nutritional status of malnourished patients with an active Crohn's disease by nutritional therapy has been established. For practical reasons two questions have to be answered: when is nutritional therapy indicated and how does it compare with medical and surgical therapy?

When is nutritional therapy indicated in active Crohn's disease?

Clearly the strongest indication for nutritional therapy in the acute phase of Crohn's disease is the treatment of nutritional deficiencies. This is quite obvious in children with growth retardation. In this situation nutritional therapy is the only successful treatment which treats malnutrition and inflammation of the intestine at once.

The second indication for nutritional therapy in patients with active Crohn's disease is preoperative treatment. It can be shown that malnutrition increases the number of postoperative complications in Crohn's patients[37,38] as well as in other surgical patients. This malnutrition can easily be treated by preoperative nutritional therapy. Müller *et al.*[29] showed, in a group of very sick Crohn's patients who were too sick to be operated on, that preoperative parenteral nutrition improved the condition of the patients so far that they could be operated electively.

Furthermore, the question arises as to whether nutritional therapy could be used instead of medical therapy or surgical therapy especially when it is considered that the majority of Crohn's patients are young and that long-term treatment with corticosteroids might have severe side effects, while frequent resections, on the other hand, might eventually lead to a short bowel syndrome.

Some investigators have used nutritional therapy for treatment of enterocutaneous fistulae. The results, however, are quite controversial. While some groups saw a closure of 70% of enterocutaneous fistulae others describe only 10% closures[23,39] and these closures are usually only temporary. Our own experience is that nutritional therapy, regardless of whether it is parenteral or enteral, is not successful as a treatment of enterocutaneous fistulae.

How does nutritional therapy compare to medical and surgical therapy?

Table 4.3 gives the overall success rates of nutritional therapy in the treatment of the acute phase of Crohn's disease. Despite the large number of studies an exact assessment of the value of nutritional therapy is difficult because of the design of most of them. Unfortunately no research has compared nutritional therapy with placebo therefore it could only be compared with the placebo groups of studies concerned with medical therapy. There are also very few randomized trials of the effect of nutritional therapy. From Table 4.3 it can be seen that the percentage of patients successfully treated with nutritional therapy as the sole treatment of the acute phase of Crohn's disease varies from study to study – since most were neither prospective nor randomized they do not allow a comparison between the effectiveness of nutritional therapy and other forms of treatment. In the only randomized study directly comparing medical treatment and nutritional therapy, medical treatment was significantly more effective with regard both to the number of patients and the time needed to reach remission[35].

Another important question concerns the long-term effect of both forms of treatment. Comparing different studies in this respect, it appears that the length of time elapsing until recurrence is quite similar regardless of whether remission was achieved by medical or nutritional therapy. More difficult is the comparison, with regard to the long-term effect, between nutritional therapy and surgical treatment since in most instances the two groups of patients are not comparable. The question rather arises as to whether, for some patients who had to be operated in earlier times, the operation might have been avoided by nutritional therapy. This is true certainly in some instances with very sick patients for whom nutritional therapy might have replaced the need for an acute surgical intervention, carrying a high risk, to elective surgery with much lower risk[29]. Patients with severe stenosis and ileus can also be treated successfully by parenteral nutrition and elective surgery can be performed later with the patient in relatively good condition. No direct comparison between the long-term effect of surgical resection and nutritional therapy has been made, however; one report used historical controls which showed that patients had fewer recurrences after surgical resections than after nutritional therapy[29].

From a practical point of view, it would be most helpful to be able to predict which patient will profit from nutritional therapy and which will not. Several attempts have been made to analyse the reaction of subgroups of Crohn's patients to nutritional therapy. The results however are controversial[30,35]. Some research showed that patients with disease of the colon do not react as well as patients with small bowel disease[30]. These data however could not be confirmed in another study[35]. At present it cannot be predicted in which patients nutritional therapy will be effective and in which not. However, patients with very severe disease seem to react less favourably than do patients with less severe disease[35].

The question was raised whether nutritional therapy is only a symptomatic therapy and whether inflammation is really reduced by this form of treatment. Again no reports document changes of the intestinal mucosa after any kind of treatment for the acute phase of Crohn's disease. However, we have performed a study measuring not only nutritional parameters but also acute phase proteins in the plasma of patients with Crohn's disease before, during and after nutritional therapy. We could show that plasma levels of acute phase reactants fell significantly during nutritional therapy and further normalized after the cessation of treatment[40]. This clearly indicates that inflammation is reduced by nutritional therapy.

NUTRITIONAL TREATMENT OF MALNUTRITION IN INACTIVE CROHN'S DISEASE

Frequently patients with Crohn's disease develop malnutrition even if the disease is inactive[20]. This malnutrition may be due to reduced oral intake, impaired intestinal absorption or increased gastrointestinal losses. Attempts to motivate patients simply to increase their food intake have not succeeded; however the addition of formula diets to the normal food has significantly increased nutritional intake of Crohn's patients over long periods[41]. It is therefore recommended that polymeric diets be used to supplement oral nutrition in malnourished patients with inactive Crohn's disease.

If, due to multiple surgical resections of the intestine, a short bowel syndrome has developed, these patients have to be treated as any other patient with short bowel syndrome.

HOW SHOULD NUTRITIONAL THERAPY BE PERFORMED?

Enteral nutrition has been shown to be as effective as parenteral nutrition in the treatment of the acute phase of Crohn's disease (see Table 4.3). Since enteral nutrition is less inconvenient and has fewer complications than parenteral nutrition, enteral nutrition should be preferred to parenteral nutrition in any case, if possible. Ileus, however, or very severe disease with fever above 38°C, vomiting, severe dehydration or stool volumes above 2000 ml per 24 h may still make parenteral nutrition necessary. Enteral nutrition solutions have to be infused via nasogastric or nasoduodenal tubes since the taste of these diets is too bad to allow offering them as drinking solutions. Decubital ulcers in the oesophagus used to be caused by hardening of plastic tubes from which the softeners were eluted during long-term nutrition. This can be avoided by using silicone or polyurethane tubes[42] which do not contain softeners and therefore do not harden even if they are used for several weeks. Constant pump infusion causes less complications than bolus infusion[43]. The location of the tip of the tube in the stomach or the duodenum seems to be less important. Usually it is easier to place the tip in the stomach. However, if one uses elemental diets the patient might experience a bad taste due to gastro-oesophageal reflux. This can be avoided by putting the tube into the duodenum. Most authors use elemental diets for enteral nutrition in Crohn's disease, even if it has yet to be shown that there is an advantage over polymeric diets with respect to absorption and clinical symptoms[44,45]. However, using α_1-antitrypsin excretion in the stool as a parameter of intestinal inflammation it has been shown that this was lower with elemental diets than with polymeric diets[46]. Starter regimens, with very slow infusion rates for the first few days and diluted nutrition solutions, do not appear to be as necessary as was initially believed[42]. However, it might be wise to increase the infusion rate slowly over 2 or 3 days to the intended rate in order to avoid complications. We start[47] with 20 ml h^{-1} and increase by 20 ml h^{-1} 12-hourly to reach the final rate of 100–120 ml h^{-1}. The upper limit of the infusion rate is set by two reactions. On the one hand, the upper limit of the absorptive capacity of the intestine may be reached and diarrhoea may occur. This clearly indicates that the infusion rate has to be reduced. On the other hand, reflux from the duodenum into the stomach increases with increasing infusion rate into the duodenum. This reflux limits the infusion rate to about 120 ml h^{-1}.

Care has to be taken to select a complete balanced diet which contains all nutritionally necessary substrates in a balanced relation. Since Crohn's patients may have multiple nutritional deficiencies, a complete diet is always preferable to supplements which do not contain everything necessary for nutrition. The same is true for parenteral nutrition. It is not useful to infuse only energy or nitrogen; one has to use a complete diet containing all necessary macro- and micronutrients. The amount of nutrition solution infused can be calculated by the estimated energy expenditure of the patient. Energy expenditure in patients with Crohn's disease is not significantly elevated[48] compared to healthy controls. Therefore it can be calculated using routine formulas. In malnourished patients it is useful to infuse 150–175% of energy expenditure. This amount allows protein synthesis and lipogenesis.

If parenteral nutrition is necessary for a patient, it has to be infused via a central venous catheter since the osmolarity of solutions used for total parenteral nutrition is too high for peripheral infusion. Routine formulations of parenteral nutrition solutions can be used for patients with Crohn's disease and no special controls are needed. However, in some patients pathological liver tests will be noted during the first weeks of parenteral nutrition[49,50]. Elevations of bilirubin and alkaline phosphatase have been described as well as of transaminases. Usually these changes are mild, self-limited and do not require special treatment. In liver biopsies done in some of these patients only unspecific changes and mild steatosis have been seen[50]. The cause of these changes is unknown. In some instances, however, good effects of metronidazole on the cholestasis have been described[49].

No clear statement can be given about the time necessary for nutritional therapy in the acute phase of Crohn's disease. Most authors use nutritional therapy for about 4 weeks. If one uses the Crohn's disease activity index (CDAI) as an indicator, nutritional therapy can be finished as soon as the CDAI is below 150. Early recurrences within the first days after cessation of nutritional therapy have not been described. For preoperative nutrition, parameters of the nutritional status are to be used as indicators of successful treatment. Plasma proteins, such as cholinesterase and albumin, as well as the red cell count are the most important parameters. Nutritional therapy of less than 10 days does not lead to a significant improvement of the nutritional status, however[47].

No research has been directed to answer the question of how to proceed in patients who do not react adequately to nutritional therapy. Additional medical treatment as well as surgical treatment should be considered, of course. However, the lack of any controlled study means the decision will have to be made according to the actual clinical situation.

CONCLUSIONS

Although appropriate medical and surgical treatment is of prime importance in the therapy of Crohn's disease, there is also evidence for a significant role for nutritional therapy in the management of patients with this disease. Many studies document a significant positive effect of nutritional therapy in patients with active Crohn's disease. Data indicate that in such patients both parenteral nutrition and enteral nutrition have supportive value particularly in the treatment of malnutrition, intestinal obstruction related to stenosis, and short bowel syndrome. Improvement of the nutritional status, however, is but one important benefit of nutritional therapy in these patients. Although so far there has only been one controlled study comparing the effects of nutritional therapy with drug treatment on disease activity in the acute phase of Crohn's disease, this indicated that, at least in some patients, nutritional therapy may also be useful as a primary treatment of the disease. Furthermore, there is evidence that supplementary nutritional therapy can improve the nutritional status of malnourished patients with inactive Crohn's disease, though no beneficial effects of plain dietary treatment of patients with inactive Crohn's disease have so far been convincingly demonstrated. As the cause and pathogenesis of Crohn's disease are still unknown, and speculations about a possible causal relationship between the intake of certain nutrients and the onset of Crohn's disease could not be substantiated, no specific dietary recommendations can be made aiming at the reduction of the incidence of Crohn's disease in general.

REFERENCES

1. Mayberry, J.F. and Rhodes, J. (1984). Epidemiological aspects of Crohn's disease: a review of the literature. *Gut*, **25**, 886–99
2. Acheson, E.D. (1960). The distribution of ulcerative colitis and regional enteritis in United States veterans with particular reference to the Jewish religion. *Gut*, **1**, 291–3
3. Lorenz-Meyer, H. and Brandes, J.W. (1983). Gibt es eine diätetische Behandlung des Morbus Crohn in der Remission? *Dtsch. Med. Wschr.*, **108**, 595–7
4. Martini, G.A. and Brandes, J.W. (1976). Increased consumption of refined carbohydrates in patients with Crohn's disease. *Klin. Wschr.*, **54**, 367
5. Miller, B., Fevers, F., Rhobeck, R. *et al.* (1976). Zuckerkonsum bei Patienten mit Morbus Crohn. *Verh. Dtsch. Ges. Inn. Med.*, **82**, 922
6. James, A.H. (1977). Breakfast and Crohn's disease. *Br. Med. J.*, **1**, 943
7. Rawcliffe, P.M. and Truelove, S.C. (1978). Breakfast and Crohn's disease. II. *Br. Med. J.*, **2**, 539
8. Thornton, J.R., Emmet, P.M. and Heaton, K.W. (1979). Diet and Crohn's disease. Characteristics of the pre-illness diet. *Br. Med. J.*, **2**, 762
9. Kasper, H. and Sommer, H. (1979). Dietary fiber and nutrient intake in Crohn's disease. *Am. J. Clin. Nutr.*, **32**, 1898
10. Mayberry, J.F., Rhodes, J. and Newcombe, R.G. (1980). Increased sugar consumption in Crohn's disease. *Digestion*, **20**, 323
11. Silkoff, K., Hallak, A., Yegena, L. *et al.* (1980). Consumption of refined carbohydrate by patients with Crohn's disease in Tel-Aviv-Yafo. *Postgrad. Med. J.*, **36**, 842
12. Mayberry, J.F., Rhodes, J,, Allan, R. *et al.* (1981). Diet in Crohn's disease. Two studies of current and previous habits in newly diagnosed patients. *Dig. Dis. Sci.*, **26**, 444–8
13. Naujoks-Heinrich, S., Grossmann, E., Gottschalk, S. *et al.* (1982). Dietary habits in Crohn's disease. *Second Symposium on Crohn's Disease*, Hemmenhofen, 1982

14. Järnerot, G., Järnmark, I. and Nilsson, K. (1983). Consumption of refined sugar by patients with Crohn's disease, ulcerative colitis, or irritable bowel syndrome. *Scand. J. Gastroenterol.*, **18**, 999–1002
15. Guthy, E. (1983). Ätiologie des Morbus Crohn. Was spricht für Fette als mögliche Ursache? *Dtsch. Med. Wschr.*, **108**, 1729–33
16. Brandes, J.W. and Lorenz-Meyer, H. (1981). Zuckerfreie Diät: Eine neue Perspektive zur Behandlung des Morbus Crohn. Eine randomisierte kontrollierte Studie. *Z. Gastroenterol.*, **19**, 1–12
17. Ritchie, J.K., Wadsworth, J., Lennard-Jones, J.E. *et al.* (1987). Controlled multicentre therapeutic trial of an unrefined carbohydrate, fibre rich diet in Crohn's disease. *Br. Med. J.*, **295**, 517–20
18. Jones, V.A., Workman, E., Freeman, A.H. *et al.* (1985). Crohn's disease: Maintenance of remission by diet. *Lancet*, **2**, 177–80
19. Jones, V.A. (1987). Comparison of total parenteral nutrition and elemental diet in induction of remission of Crohn's disease. Long-term maintenance of remission by personalized food exclusion diets. *Dig. Dis. Sci.*, **32**, 100S–107S
20. Driscoll, R.H. and Rosenberg, I.H. (1978). Total parenteral nutrition in inflammatory bowel disease. *Med. Clin. North Am.*, **62**,185–201
21. Morin, C.L., Roulet, M., Roy, C.C. *et al.* (1980). Continuous elemental enteral alimentation in children with Crohn's disease and growth failure. *Gastroenterology*, **79**, 1205–10
22. Peters, H. (1976). Parenteral-perorale Kombinationsbehandlung von Morbus Crohn und Colitis ulcerosa. *Infusionstherapie*, **3**, 222–6
23. Fromm, H., Gebel, M., Schroeter, U. (1978). Zur Behandlung des Morbus Crohn im akuten Stadium. *Dtsch. Med. Wschr.*, **9**, 377–80
24. Dickinson, R.J., Ashton, M.G., Axon, A.T.R. *et al.* (1980). Controlled trial of intravenous hyperalimentation and total bowel rest as an adjunct of the routine therapy of acute colitis. *Gastroenterology*, **79**, 1199–204
25. Kirschner, B.S., Klich, J.R., Kalman, S. *et al.* (1981). Reversal of growth retardation in Crohn's disease with therapy emphasizing oral nutrition restitution. *Gastroenterology*, **80**, 10–15
26. Meryn, S, Lochs, H., Rötzi, R. *et al.* (1982). Einfluss von parenteraler Ernährung auf Serumproteine bei Patienten mit Morbus Crohn. *Infusionstherapie*, **9**, 149–52
27. Morin, C.L., Roulet, M., Ray, C.C. *et al.* (1982). Continuous elemental enteral alimentation in the treatment of children and adolescents with Crohn's disease. *J. Parent. Ent. Nutr.*, **6**, 194–9
28. Lochs, H., Meryn, S., Marosi, L. *et al.* (1983). Has total bowel rest a beneficial effect in the treatment of Crohn's disease? *Clin. Nutr.*, **2**, 61–74
29. Müller, J.M., Keller, H.W., Erasmi, H. *et al.* (1983). Total parenteral nutrition as the sole therapy in Crohn's disease – a prospective study. *Br. J. Surg.*, **70**, 40–3
30. Lochs, H., Egger-Schödl, M., Schuh, R. *et al.* (1984). Is tube feeding with elemental diets a primary therapy of Crohn's disease? *Klin. Wschr.*, **237**, 1–5
31. Ostro, M.J., Greenberg, G.R. and Jeejeebhoy, K.N. (1985). Total parenteral nutrition and complete bowel rest in the management of Crohn's disease. *J. Parent. Ent. Nutr.*, **9**, 280–7
32. Lerebours, E., Messing, B., Chevalier, B. *et al.* (1986). An evaluation of total parenteral nutrition in the management of steroid-dependent and steroid-resistant patients with Crohn's disease. *J. Parent. Ent. Nutr.*, **10**, 274–8
33. Rabast, U. and Heskamp, R. (1986). Adjuvante Therapie mit Formeldiäten bei chronisch-entzündlichen Darmerkrankungen. *Dtsch. Med. Wschr.*, **111**, 293–7
34. Greenberg, G.R., Fleming, C.R., Jeejeebhoy, K.N. *et al.* (1988). Controlled trial of bowel rest and nutritional support in the management of Crohn's disease. *Gut*, **29**, 1309–15
35. Lochs, H., Steinhardt, H.J., Klaus-Wenz, B. *et al.* (1988). Enteral nutrition *versus* drug treatment for the acute phase of Crohn's disease: Results of the European Co-operative Crohn's Disease Study IV. *Gastroenterology*, **94**, A267
36. Motil, K.J., Grand, R.J., Matthews, D.E. *et al.* (1982). Whole body leucine metabolism in adolescents with Crohn's disease and growth failure during nutritional supplementation. *Gastroenterology*, **82**, 1359–68

37. Higgens, C.S., Keighley, M.R.B. and Allan, R.N. (1984). Impact of preoperative weight loss and body composition changes on postoperative outcome in surgery for inflammatory bowel disease. *Gut*, **25**, 732–6
38. Lindon, K.D., Fleming, C.R. and Ilstrup, D.M. (1985). Preoperative nutritional status and other factors that influence surgical outcome in patients with Crohn's disease. *Mayo Clin. Proc.*, **60**, 393–6
39. MacFayden, B.V., Jr., Dudrick, S.J. and Ruberg, R.L. (1973). Management of gastrointestinal fistulas with parenteral hyperalimentation. *Surgery*, **74**, 100–5
40. Meryn, S., Lochs, H., Pamperl, H. *et al.* (1983). Influence of parenteral nutrition on serum levels of proteins in patients with Crohn's disease. *J. Parent. Ent. Nutr.*, **7**, 553–6
41. Harries, A.D., Danis, V., Heatley, R.V. *et al.* (1983). Controlled trial of supplemented oral nutrition in Crohn's disease. *Lancet*, **1**, 887–90
42. Jones, B.J.M. (1986). Enteral feeding: techniques of administration. *Gut*, **27**, (S1), 47–50
43. Jones, B.J.M., Payne, S. and Silk, D.B.A. (1980). Indications for pump-assisted enteral feeding. *Lancet*, **2**, 1057–8
44. Silk, D.B.A. (1986). Diet formulation and choice of enteral diet. *Gut*, **27**, (S1), 40–6
45. Moriarty, K.J., Hegarty, J.E., Fairclough, P.D. *et al.* (1985). Relative nutritional value of whole protein, hydrolysed protein and free amino acids in man. *Gut*, **26**, 694–9
46. Steinhardt, H.J., Payer, E., Henn, B. *et al.* (1987). Beeinflusst die Proteinkomponente von Formuladiäten die Stickstoffabsorption beim Morbus Crohn? *Z. Gastroenterol.*, **8**, 573
47. Lochs, H. (1988). Infusions- und Ernährungstherapie bei entzündlichen Darmerkrankungen. In: Reissigl, H. (ed.) *Handbuch der Infusionstherapie und klinischen Ernährung*, Band IV, pp. 169–84
48. Chan, A.T.H., Fleming, C.R., O'Fallon, W.M. *et al.* (1986). Estimated versus measured basal energy requirement in patients with Crohn's disease. *Gastroenterology*, **91**, 75–8
49. Matuchansky, C. (1986). Parenteral nutrition in inflammatory bowel disease. *Gut*, **27**, (S1), 81–4
50. Bengoa, J.M., Hanauer, S.B., Sitrin, M.D. *et al.* (1985). Pattern and prognosis of liver function test abnormalities during parenteral nutrition in inflammatory bowel disease. *Hepatology*, **5**, 79–84

5
Pathophysiology and treatment of extraintestinal symptoms in Crohn's disease

J. SCHÖLMERICH

INTRODUCTION

Extraintestinal symptoms are common in several diseases of the intestinal tract[1–5]. In some cases these symptoms determine the course of the disease and are sometimes difficult to treat. This is particularly the case with Crohn's disease and ulcerative colitis. Two types of extraintestinal symptoms can be distinguished: extraintestinal manifestations; and extraintestinal complications. The pathogenesis of the manifestations is not definitively clear. Where external organs such as skin, eyes and joints are affected, diagnosis is easier. In contrast, the pathogenesis of complications is mostly known, but particularly deficiency syndromes have a slow course and are difficult to diagnose. Treatment of manifestations is based on anti-inflammatory drugs as in the underlying bowel disease while complications can be treated causally due to the known pathogenesis.

EXTRAINTESTINAL MANIFESTATIONS

The extraintestinal manifestations of chronic inflammatory bowel disease in most instances affect joints, skin and eyes but can also be related to a multiplicity of other organs. The occurrence of these extraintestinal manifestations correlates with the activity of the bowel disease although they can be the initial symptom[2,6–8].

Description and incidence

Greenstein, in 1976, analysed a large number of patients with chronic inflammatory bowel disease with respect to the incidence of extraintestinal manifestations[1]. In addition, the two large multicentre trials of treatment of

Crohn's disease from the United States[9] and from Europe (L.Hoj, unpublished), both including about 500 patients, analysed the prevalence and incidence of extraintestinal manifestations. It can be estimated that 60–80% of all patients with Crohn's disease will present during their lifetime with one or the other extraintestinal manifestation. The frequency is dependent on the localization of the disease. Patients with colonic involvement are more often affected than those with small bowel disease only (Table 5.1). If the studies mentioned above[1–3,9] are taken together, the frequency of joint inflammation (monoarthritis or polyarthritis) is 20–35%, skin abnormalities (erythema nodosum, pyoderma gangrenosum) occur in 5–28% and eye lesions (iridocyclitis, episcleritis and uveitis) in 4–8%.

Disturbed pulmonary function is more frequent than is generally known since about 50% of all patients demonstrate abnormal lung function tests when they are systematically assessed[10]. These abnormalities only rarely produce clinical symptoms. However, in some instances alveolitis and fibrosis-like affections have been found[11]. Abnormalities of the liver are also relatively common and can occur in up to 50% of patients during the course of the disease[3,12–15]. This spectrum includes sinusoidal dilatation, granulomatous hepatatis, pericholangitis and primary sclerosing cholangitis with liver cirrhosis[12,13]. Obviously primary sclerosing cholangitis in some cases is asymptomatic and will only be detected with endoscopic retrograde cholangiopancreatography (ERCP)[15].

Further rare manifestations include pancreatitis[16], vasculitis[17], pericarditis and myocarditis[18], autoimmune haemolytic anaemia, thromboembolic diseases[17], and amyloidosis[19]. The prevalence of all these rare lesions is below 1%[3].

Table 5.1 Frequency of extraintestinal manifestations in Crohn's disease

	Colitis (%)	*Ileocolitis* (%)	*Ileitis* (%)
Erythema nodosum	15	8	4
Pyoderma gangrenosum	2	1	1
Polyarthritis	15	10	6
Monoarthritis	17	11	5
Eye lesions	13	4	1

Source: Greenstein *et al.* (1976)[1]

Pathogenesis

Most of these extraintestinal manifestations occur with several different diseases of the gastrointestinal tract. The finding that the risk of developing such associated manifestations, in particular sacroileitis or ankylosing spondylitis, is increased in patients with an expression of HLA-B27 and other such associations supports a genetic predisposition for the occurrence of extraintestinal manifestations. This is further supported by the fact that the occurrence of these lesions associated with HLA-B27 is not correlated with the activity of the disease. The exact role of such genetic associations for the occurrence or persistence of extraintestinal manifestations is not known, however. In patients with chronic inflammatory bowel disease an increased permeability of the intestinal mucosa during active exacerbations of the disease has been found. Furthermore, an increased permeability has also been demonstrated in patients and in their not-diseased relatives more recently[20]. Increased absorption of several antigens could, therefore, play a role in the initiation and permeation of local and extraintestinal abnormal immunological reactions. The effects of the gut-associated immune system have been discussed[6]. Several findings support a role for circulating immune complexes in the pathogenesis of extraintestinal manifestations. Immune

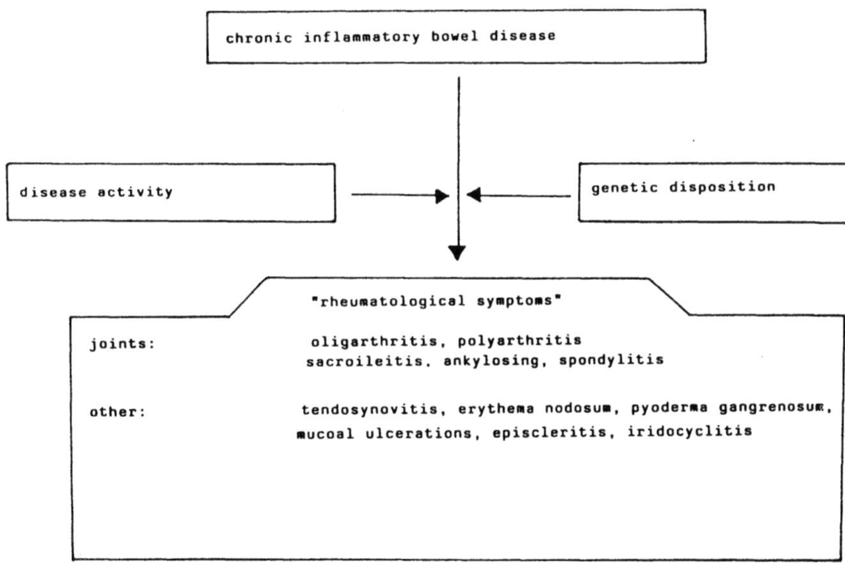

Figure 5.1 Pathophysiology of extraintestinal manifestations in chronic inflammatory bowel disease. Modified from Hermann *et al.* (1988)[6]

complex nephritis has been demonstrated in a patient with Crohn's disease[21]. Other immune mediated diseases such as primary biliary cirrhosis have been found in association with inflammatory bowel disease[22]. A general scheme for the pathogenesis of extraintestinal manifestations in chronic inflammatory bowel diseases is given in Figure 5.1.

Table 5.2 Side effects of sulphasalazine

Organ	*Symptoms*
Bone marrow	Aplastic anaemia Agranulocytosis Thrombopenia Leukopenia
Erythrocytes	Haemolytic anaemia
Skin	Erythema Exfoliative dermatitis Alopecia
Eyes	Episcleritis
General reactions	Fever Arthralgia
Heart	Myocarditis Pericarditis
Lung	Fibrosing alveolitis
Sensory organs	Taste disturbances Ear abnormalities
Liver	'Hepatitis'

Source: Miller (1980)[23]

It is of some importance that drugs which are used in the treatment of chronic inflammatory bowel disease can induce a significant number of the symptoms discussed above (Table 5.2)[3,23]. Therefore differentiation of the side effects of drugs and extraintestinal manifestations is necessary in individual cases.

Several pathogenetic principles with respect to the frequent abnormalities of the hepatobiliary system are under discussion. In particular, bacteria in the portal vein, malabsorption and, finally, a similar mechanism as in the other extraintestinal manifestations have been proposed[13,14]. Several groups failed to demonstrate abnormalities of the bile acid spectrum in the portal vein and relations to liver abnormalities in chronic inflammatory bowel disease[24,25]. Recently, autoantibodies against bowel mucosa cross-reacting with antigens of the portal tract have been described in sera of patients with inflammatory bowel disease[26]. Probably several mechanisms are involved in the pathogenesis of hepatobiliary abnormalities in chronic inflammatory bowel disease.

Treatment

The treatment of most extraintestinal manifestations is similar to that of the underlying disease. Anti-inflammatory drugs are prefered, steriods in particular[2]. It is not exactly known if the application of sulphasalazine is effective in treating the joint lesions. It has been suggested that the sulphapyridine component of the molecule may be the active component for synovial inflammation[2]. It has to be mentioned that the application of non-steroidal anti-inflammatory drugs may be associated with exacerbations of Crohn's disease and may even simulate this disease[27]. Skin lesions are generally treated by decreasing the activity of the underlying inflammatory bowel disease. Topical hydrocortisone treatment is only rarely necessary in erythema nodosum but appropriate in pyoderma gangrenosum. The use of immunosuppressive agents in the treatment of resistant pyoderma gangrenosum has been advocated[2]. The ocular manifestations are treated by a reduction of the inflammation in the bowel along with the use of local ocular hydrocortisone solutions.

Treatment of hepatobiliary abnormalities is difficult and not equivocal. Neither steroids nor D-penicillamine have been found to be effective[28]. Recent studies have shown, however, that the course of primary sclerosing cholangitis, diagnosed using invasive diagnostic schedules including ERCP, is relatively benign (Figure 5.2). Studies using methotrexate or colchicine are under way but no definitive results are available. Liver transplantation remains the only curative treatment so far. Most of the other rare manifestations are also treated with oral steroids. In particular, pleuropericarditis and lung affections are responsive to such treatment[3,11,29]. Associated pancreatitis has been described as responding to local resection of the bowel segment involved[30]. There is no known treatment for amyloidosis. The thromboembolic complications are treated with the usual anticoagulant drugs. However, fibrinolysis is contraindicated in active bowel disease.

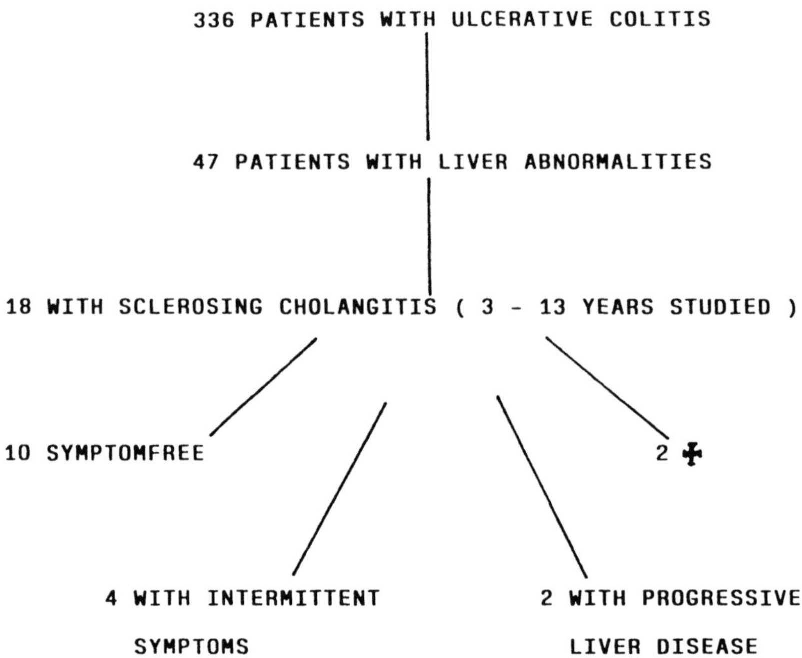

Figure 5.2 Frequency and course of primary sclerosing cholangitis in patients with ulcerative colitis. Taken from Schrumpf *et al.* (1982)[15]

Exclusion of the side effects of drugs used in the treatment of bowel disease has to be the first step in all attempts to treat extraintestinal manifestations of inflammatory bowel disease.

EXTRAINTESTINAL COMPLICATIONS

Extraintestinal complications in chronic inflammatory bowel disease are caused in most instances by a decreased or, rarely, increased amount of exogenous substances in the organism as a consequence of a disturbed bowel function[3,4]. Deficiencies of vitamins, trace elements, protein, and bile acids, and increased resorption of oxalate are the most important abnormalities (Table 5.3).

Table 5.3 Extraintestinal complications of Crohn's disease

Complications	*Symptoms*
Vitamin deficiency	Osteomalacia Muscle atrophy Night blindness Inner ear deafness Taste disturbances Hyperkeratosis Anaemia
Trace element deficiency	Anaemia Osteomalacia Growth retardation Disturbed wound healing Oligospermia Immune deficiency
Protein deficiency	Oedema Transport protein deficiency
Hyperoxaluria, water loss	Renal calculi
Bile acid deficiency	Gallstones

Deficiency syndromes: description, incidence and symptoms

Deficiencies of vitamins, electrolytes, and trace elements are in general due to the dysfunction of the small bowel. It therefore occurs more frequently in patients with Crohn's disease than in those with other inflammatory diseases, in particular ulcerative colitis.

Reports of the frequency of nutritional deficiencies in patients with Crohn's disease demonstrate anaemia of several causes in 50–70%. The anaemia is not always correlated with the activity of the disease. Abnormalities of bone metabolism which are caused mostly by vitamin D and/or calcium deficiency are found in up to 60% of patients with Crohn's disease when patients are routinely assessed[31–33]. Pathological or borderline absorption of vitamin B_{12} is observed in up to 60% of patients with Crohn's disease (Figure 5.3). Signs of vitamin C deficiency are found in up to 37% of patients[34]. Deficiency of zinc is mostly found in patients with active Crohn's disease[35], the frequency depends on the technique used for the assessment[36,37]. Deficiency of vitamin A is also related to activity of the disease[35,38] but may also be observed in patients with inactive disease and extensive ileal resection. Zinc and vitamin A deficiency seem to be more

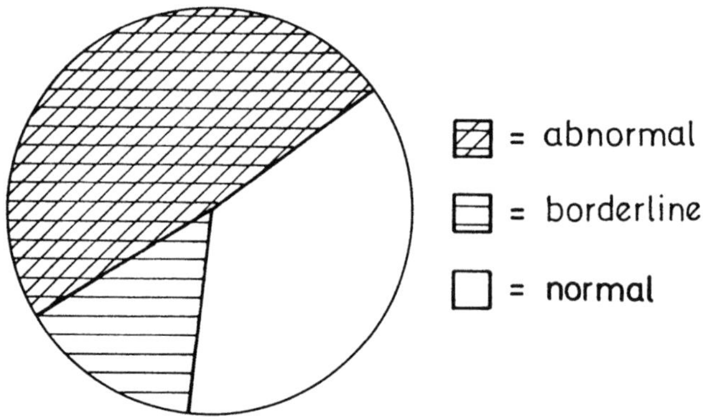

Figure 5.3 Vitamin B_{12} absorption in an unselected group of patients with Crohn's disease

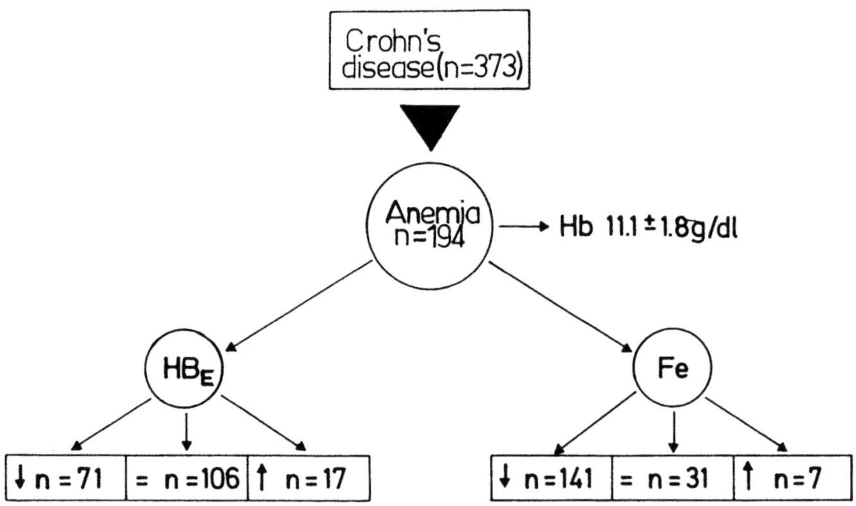

Figure 5.4 Different forms of anaemia in patients with Crohn's disease. Taken from Balzer *et al.* (1984)[40]

common in younger patients[39]. No information is available with regard to other rare vitamins.

The occurrence of one or a combination of these deficiencies can result in a variety of symptoms (Table 5.3). In particular anaemia and osteomalacia are of importance for the prognosis and life quality of the patient. Anaemia can be due to several deficiencies (Figure 5.4)[40]. Several sensory dysfunctions such as dark blindness, disturbed taste acuity, inner ear deafness and other abnormalities can be found using appropriate techniques. It has been suggested that taste abnormalities can influence malnutrition[41]. Growth retardation as sign of protein and zinc deficiency[39,42] and a disturbed sexual development are of paramount importance in children. Disturbed spermiogenesis[43], coagulation defects and delayed wound healing have been described but are rare. It is not known if the disturbed immune response is at least in part due to deficiencies.

Pathogenesis of deficiencies

The pathogenesis of the different deficiencies is variable. Increased consumption of iron, zinc and folic acid has been found. In contrast, increased loss is a cause of iron, potassium, sodium and calcium deficiency. Disturbed absorption is probably the cause of the deficiency of other substances. Interactions between different deficiencies have to be considered (Figure 5.5)[4]. Side effects of the drugs used in the treatment of inflammatory bowel disease can be a further cause of deficiency states. Prednisolone, as well as sulphasalazine and, for obvious reasons, the bile acid binder cholestyramine,

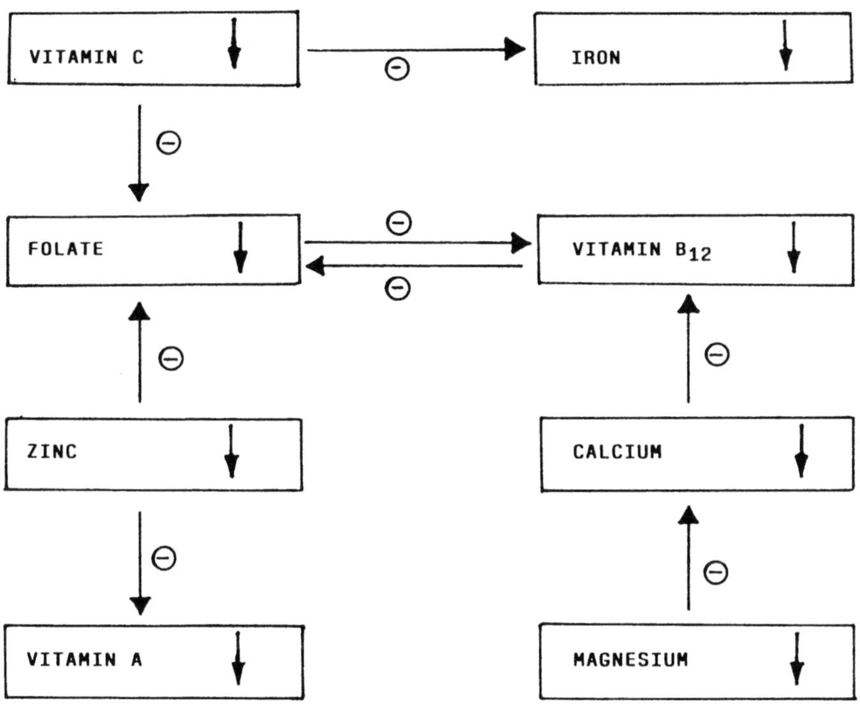

Figure 5.5 Interactions of deficiencies of trace elements and vitamins

can influence several mechanisms via the metabolism of vitamins and trace elements (Table 5.4). A reduction of folic acid absorption with sulphasalazine treatment and the increased consumption of vitamin C and vitamin B_6 with prednisone treatment have been described[4]. Several symptoms of deficiency such as disturbed spermiogenesis can also be explained as drug side effects[43]. This might also be the case for the taste abnormalities[41,44]. Finally, resections of individual parts of the bowel can play a significant role in the development of deficiency states. This is in particular true for fat malabsorption and for vitamin B_{12} deficiency with resection of the terminal ileum[45].

Table 5.4 Influence of drugs used in the treatment of inflammatory bowel disease on deficiencies

Prednisone	–	zinc ↓	(loss)
	–	vitamin C ↓	(consumption)
	–	vitamin B_6 ↓	(consumption)
	–	vitamin D ↓	(antagonism)
Sulphasalazine	–	folate ↓	(absorption ↓)
	–	iron ↓	(haemolysis ↓)
Cholestyramine	–	vitamin D ↓	(absorption ↓)
	–	vitamin B_{12} ↓	(absorption ↓)
	–	iron ↓	(absorption ↓)

Diagnosis of deficiency states

Simple laboratory tests are sufficient for the detection of most deficiency states (Table 5.5). However, some symptoms such as osteomalacia can only be diagnosed with more aggressive techniques[33]. In particular, computed tomography bone density measurements, bone biopsy and assessment of different vitamin D metabolites are of importance in detecting all patients with disorders of mineral and bone metabolism. For routine assessment, probably vitamin D analysis and a conventional X-ray study of the vertebral column might be sufficient. Vitamin B_{12} resorption can easily be assessed using the Schilling test. Sensory function tests are laborious and should only be made when abnormalities are suspected. Spermiography is useful in young patients with a frustrated desire for children. In children the assessment of growth age is necessary.

The assessment of serum or plasma concentrations of trace elements and vitamins does not always give enough information about deficiency states[4,33,36,37].

Table 5.5 Diagnosis of extraintestinal complications in Crohn's disease

Laboratory:	Fe, Ca, Mg, Zn Ferritin Vitamin B_{12}, folate Vitamin D_3 Alkaline phosphatase, SGOT Albumin Haemoglobin, Hb_E
Technical:	Vitamin B_{12} – absorption Vertebral column X-ray (CT-densitometry) (SeCAT-test)

Treatment of deficiencies

The treatment of diagnosed deficiency is simple and based on adequate substitution. The route of substitution has to be adapted to the expected or defined cause of the deficiency. In particular, vitamin B_{12} and fat-soluble vitamins can be substituted parenterally only when the terminal ileum is either resected or diseased to a large extent[4]. Control of substitution using serum analysis is in most instances sufficient and results in normal values in a controlled and substituted group of patients as shown in Figure 5.6. Successful treatment of taste abnormalities[44] and disturbed dark adaptation[46,47] has been reported (Figure 5.7). Manifest osteomalacia has been successfully treated with vitamin D substitution[32]. Growth retardation was improved by application of zinc[39] and a general improvement of nutrition in addition to drug treatment[39]. Anaemia can generally be improved by substitution with either iron, vitamin B_{12} or folic acid. In general, it is of major importance for the diagnosis and the treatment of deficiency states in patients with chronic inflammatory bowel disease to consider such deficiencies and to attempt diagnosis.

Cholecystolithiasis and nephrolithiasis: pathogenesis

Patients with Crohn's disease have a significantly increased frequency of gallstones and renal calculi[48,49] (Table 5.6). These abnormalities are more frequent with resection of the terminal ileum[48,50]. Gallstones are, as a rule, cholesterol stones, renal calculi consist of calcium oxalate in most cases.

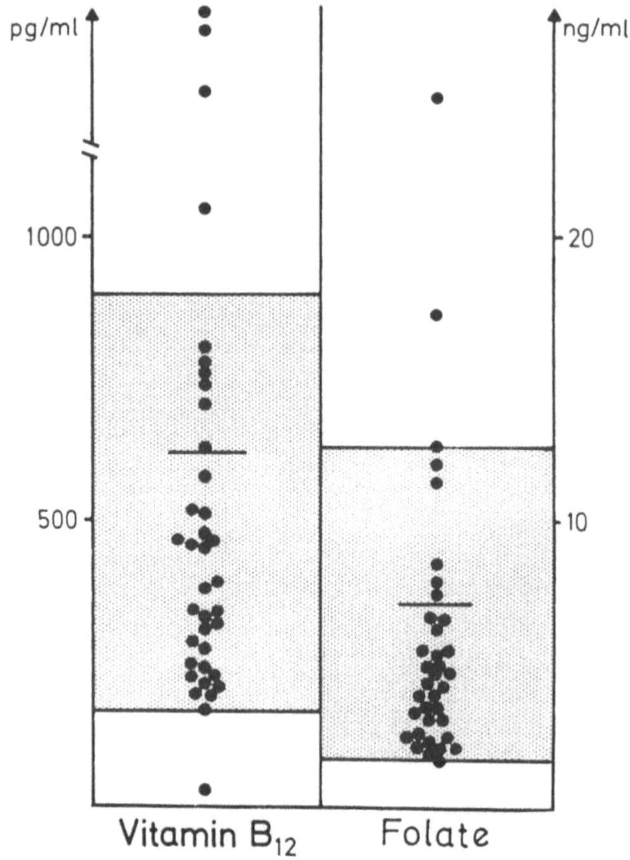

Figure 5.6 Serum concentrations of vitamin B_{12} and folate in controlled and substituted patients with Crohn's disease

Table 5.6 Ultrasound findings in 74 patients with Crohn's disease

	n	%
Gallstones	9	12.2
Cholecystectomy	5	6.8
Cholelithiasis, total	14	18.8
Renal calculi	7	9.5
Liver abnormalities	17	23.0

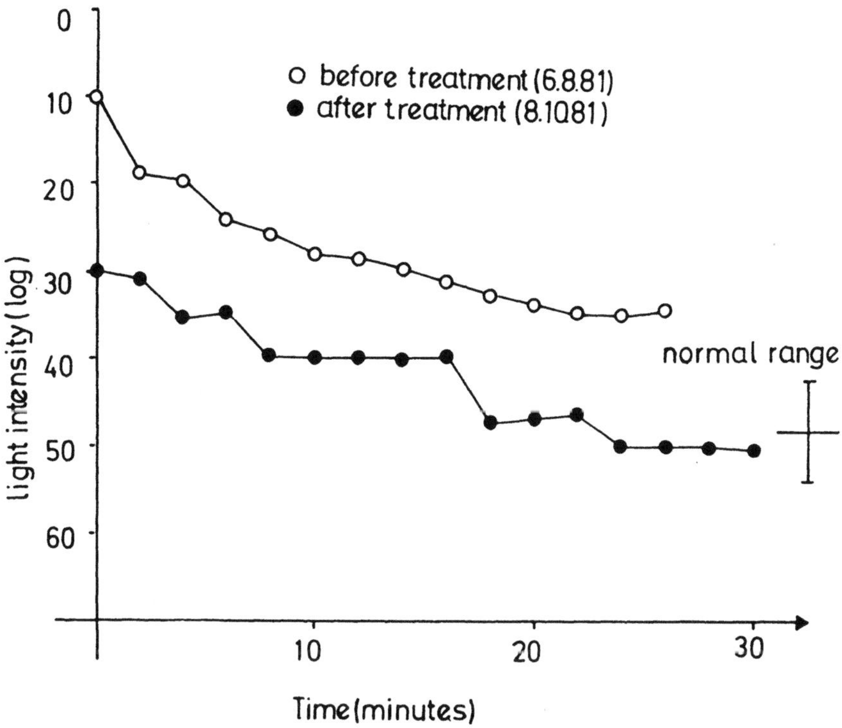

Figure 5.7 Influence of vitamin A on dark adaption in patients with Crohn's disease. Taken from Main *et al.* (1983)[46]

The increased occurrence of cholecystolithiasis and nephrolithiasis is mainly due to the disturbed enterohepatic circulation of bile acids[51]. The major part of bile acids is actively resorbed in the terminal ileum. This explains the decreased bile acid resorption in patients with Crohn's disease[52–55]. The resorption of chenodeoxycholic acid in patients without resection has been found to be only 25% of controls. Similar findings have been shown for cholic acid[52,53] (Table 5.7). The resulting increased cholesterol saturation of bile explains, at least in part, the increased risk of cholesterol gallstones in this patient group[54]. The risk is further increased in patients with resection of the terminal ileum[49,50]. It is not known if abnormal contraction or motility of gallbladder and bile ducts in these patients have an additional role.

Table 5.7 Absorption of bile acids in patients with Crohn's disease

	Chenodeoxycholate[a]	*Cholate*[a]
Controls ($n = 46$)	114 ± 7	317 ± 20
Crohn's disease without resection ($n = 8$)	29 ± 6	93 ± 18
Crohn's disease with resection ($n = 7$)	12 ± 6	91 ± 39

[a] AUC μmol per litre × min.
Source: Heumann *et al.*[52]

Table 5.8 Treatment of extraintestinal complications in Crohn's disease

(1) Gallstones	–	surgery if symptomatic
(2) Renal calculi	–	lithotripsy
(3) Stone prophylaxis	–	medium-chain triglycerides
	–	calcium
	–	reduced oxalate in diet
(4) Substitution (if deficiency)	–	vitamins: B_{12}, A, D, E, K, folate
	–	trace elements: Fe, Ca, Mg, Zn

Bile acid malabsorption is of importance in the pathogenesis of renal calculi as well. Due to the lack of bile acids, disturbed fat absorption results in an increased influx of fatty acids and decreased availability of calcium in the colon. Thus, more oxalate is available for resorption. Fatty acids and bile acids increase oxalate resorption[51,56]. In addition, endogenous synthesis of oxalate in the liver is increased due to increased catabolism of glycine in the colon[56]. Zinc and vitamin A deficiency favour crystallization of calcium oxalate in urine[56] (Figure 5.8). The risk of nephrolithiasis also increases with ileal resection[49,50]. In patients with steatorrhoea and ileal resection the risk is 26 times higher than in patients with only steatorrhoea[50].

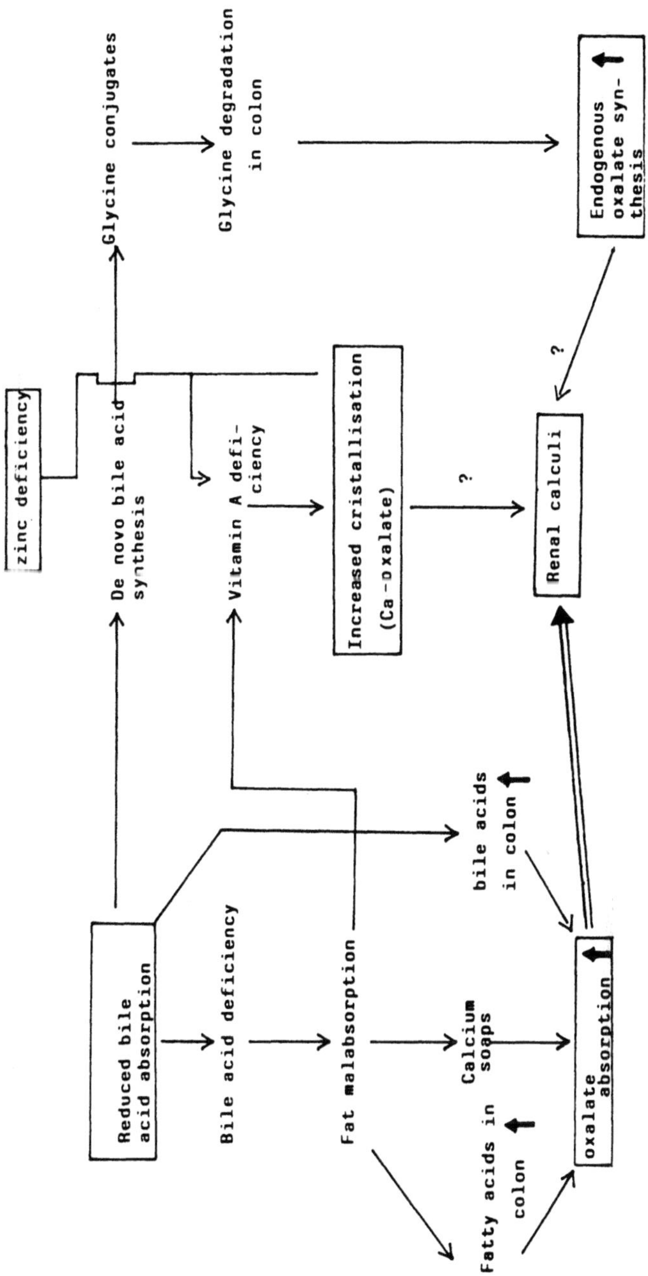

Figure 5.8 Pathophysiology of calcium-oxalate stones in patients with Crohn's disease. Modified from Müller *et al.* (1987)[56]

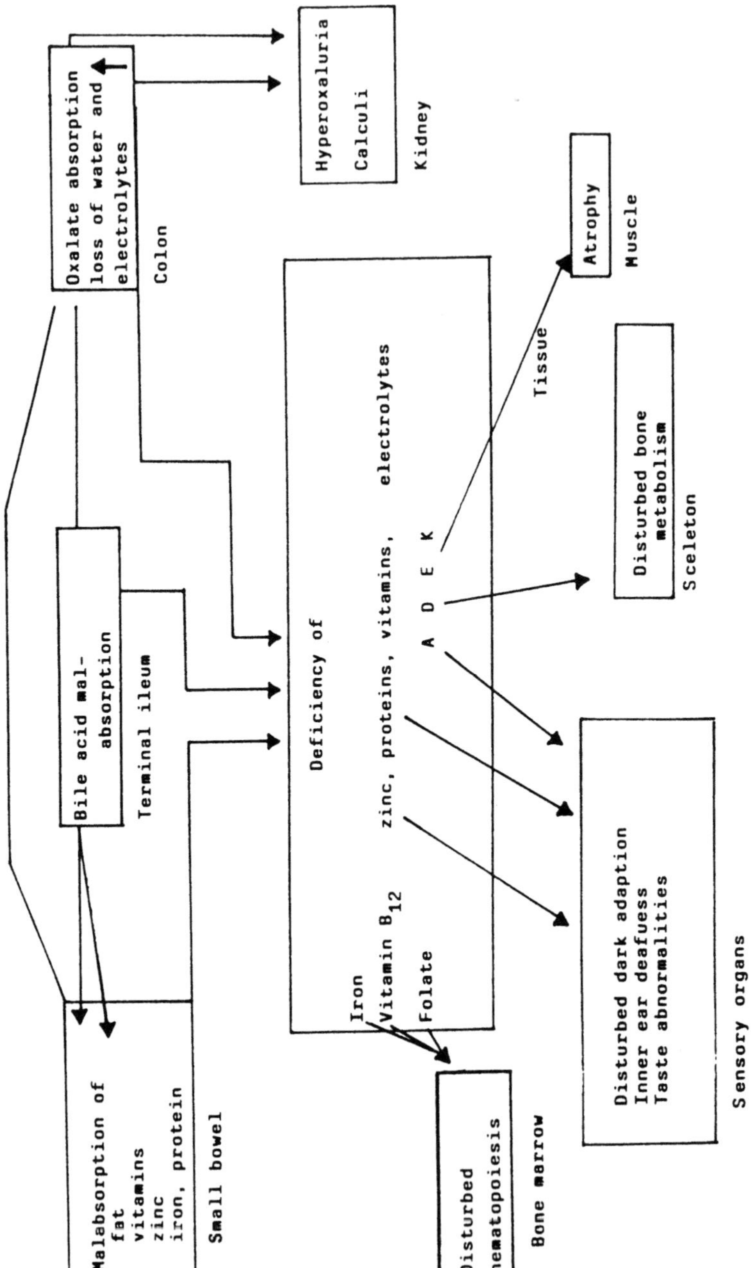

Figure 5.9 Pathophysiology of extraintestinal complications in patients with Crohn's disease

Diagnosis and treatment of cholecystolithiasis and nephrolithiasis

The occurrence of cholecystolithiasis and nephrolithiasis is easily detected by regular sonographic controls (Table 5.6). Using this technique, other extraintestinal symptoms, i.e. of the liver or the pancreas, can also be detected[49].

The treatment is similar to that in patients without inflammatory bowel disease. Asymptomatic gallstones do not deserve treatment. Symptomatic stones require cholecystectomy. Conservative methods of treatment such as oral litholysis using urso- or chenodeoxycholic acid or extracorporeal shock-wave lithotripsy are not useful in these patients since abnormal bile acid absorption prevents effective treatment. It is of importance to recognize that symptoms of cholecystolithiasis, such as acute cholecystitis, can be misinterpreted as an exacerbation of the known inflammatory bowel disease. This can result in mistaken steroid treatment and thereby aggravate symptoms.

Renal stones can be treated by several techniques. In particular extracorporeal shock-wave lithotripsy might be attempted. Several prophylactic treatments are available. The application of medium-chain triglycerides reduces fat malabsorption since these medium-chain fatty acids do not require bile acids for resorption. A reduction of oxalate in the diet as well as the application of calcium reduces the available amount of oxalate for resorption in the colon. Cholestyramine can bind bile acids, thus reducing bile acid-dependent oxalate resorption and at the same time chologenic diarrhoea (Table 5.8).

The pathogenesis of the described extraintestinal complications is complex and can be understood with a few exceptions (Figure 5.9). Diagnosis is relatively simple. Treatment includes prophylactic substitution and dietetic adaption in patients with resection or extensive disease of the terminal ileum.

MALIGNANT TUMOURS

Accumulating evidence suggests that not only in patients with ulcerative colitis but also in patients with Crohn's disease there is an increased risk of the development of intestinal and extraintestinal neoplasia[57–59]. The risk is, however, smaller than in patients with ulcerative colitis[57–59]. It is of particular interest that patients with Crohn's disease have an increased risk of perianal carcinoma and carcinoma of the lower genital tract in female patients[58] (Figure 5.10). Cholangiocarcinoma is associated with primary sclerosing cholangitis although in some instances cases of carcinoma without this association have been described[60].

Whether regular controls, such as in ulcerative colitis, are necessary and helpful in patients with Crohn's disease is not well defined. In particular, in patients with extensive disease of the colon a similar scheme of prophylactic colonoscopy seems probably appropriate. A prophylactic screening scheme for extraintestinal neoplasias has also yet to be defined.

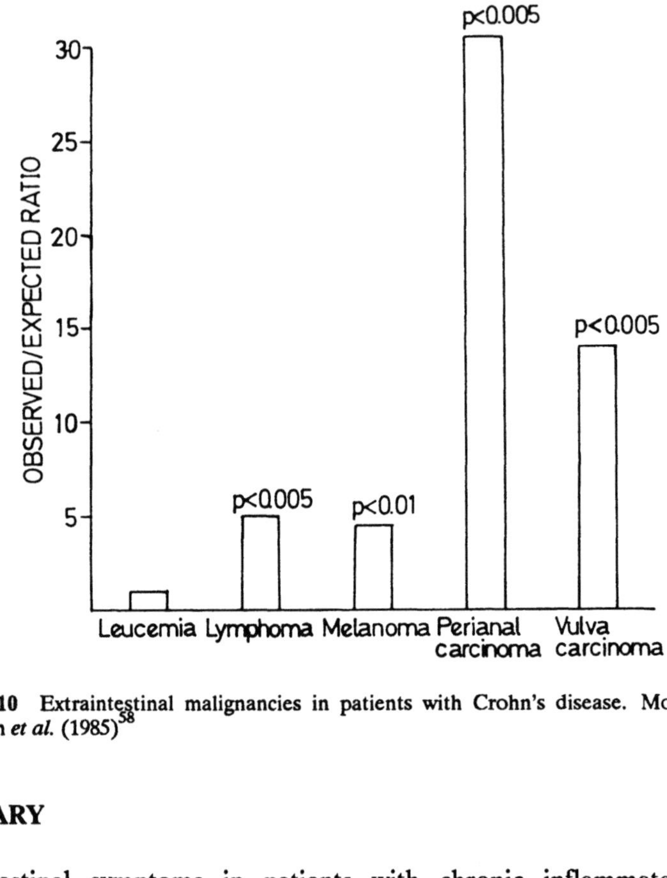

Figure 5.10 Extraintestinal malignancies in patients with Crohn's disease. Modified from Greenstein *et al.* (1985)[58]

SUMMARY

Extraintestinal symptoms in patients with chronic inflammatory bowel disease are frequent and in some instances lead to diagnosis. Extraintestinal manifestations can be distinguished from extraintestinal complications. During the course of their disease 60–80% of patients present with extraintestinal manifestations – mostly affecting joints, skin and eyes. Abnormalities of liver and lung are also common but often subclinical. Affections of other organ systems are rare. The pathogenesis of extra-intestinal manifestations is not definitively clear; a genetic predisposition exists. Probably a dysfunction of the gut-associated immune system is of importance. The treatment is basically the same as that of the underlying disease.

Extraintestinal complications are due to disturbed bowel function. Deficiency and deficiency symptoms are common and more difficult to diagnose. Substitution can successfully prevent or treat deficiencies. Anaemia and osteomalacia are of special importance since they influence prognosis and life quality. Gallstones and renal calculi are due to disturbed intrahepatic circulation of bile acids. They can be rather easily diagnosed using sonography.

Patients with Crohn's disease probably have an increased risk of intestinal and extraintestinal neoplasia. Regular controls might be of value for these patients.

REFERENCES

1. Greenstein, A.J., Janowitz, H.D. and Sachar, D.B. (1976). The extra-intestinal complications of Crohn's disease and ulcerative colitis: A study of 700 patients. *Medicine*, **55**, 401–12
2. Danzi, J.T. (1988). Extraintestinal manifestations of idiopathic inflammatory bowel disease. *Arch. Intern. Med.*, **148**, 297–302
3. Schölmerich, J., Hoppe-Seyler, P. and Gerok, W. (1986). Extraintestinale Manifestationen bei entzündlichen Darmerkrankungen. *Therapiewoche*, **36**, 520–32
4. Schölmerich, J. (1986). Vitamin- und Spurenelementmangel bei entzündlichen Darmerkrankungen. In Ewe, K. and Fahrländer, H. (eds.) *Therapie chronisch entzündlicher Darmerkrankungen*, pp. 95–107. (Schattauer: Stuttgart/New York)
5. Nord, H.J. (1987). Complications of inflammatory bowel disease. *Hosp. Pract.*, **22**, 65–82
6. Hermann, E., Mayet, E., Poralla, W.J. and Meyer zum Büschenfelde, K.H. (1988). Rheumatologische Aspekte bei Magen-Darmerkrankungen. Klinik und pathologische Aspekte. *Z. Gastroenterol.*, **26**, 137–44
7. Brackertz, D. (1987). Arthritiden bei Colitis ulcerosa und Morbus Crohn. *Z. Rheumatol.*, **46**, 14–21
8. Russel, A.S. (1988). Inflammatory bowel disease: Associated rheumatologic conditions. *Can. J. Gastroenterol.*, **2**, 117A–119A
9. Rankin, G.B., Watts, D., Melnyk, C.S. and Kelley, M.L. (1979). National co-operative Crohn's disease study: Extraintestinal manifestations and perianal complications. *Gastroenterology*, **77**, 914–20
10. Sommer, H., Schmidt, M. and Gruber, K.D. (1986). Lungenfunktionsstörungen bei Colitis ulcerosa und Morbus Crohn. *Dtsch. Med. Wschr.*, **111**, 812–5
11. Germann, P.P.-J., Schölmerich, J., Costabel, U., Guzman, J., Pausch, J. and Gerok, W. (1988). Koinzidenz von Colitis ulcerosa und Lungenfibrose – eine seltene extraintestinale Manifestation chronisch entzündlicher Darmerkrankungen? *Med. Klin.*, **83**, 461–3
12. Desmet, V.J. and Geboes, K. (1987). Liver lesions in inflammatory bowel disorders. *J. Pathol.*, **151**, 247–55
13. Christophi, C. and Hughes, E.R. (1985). Hepatobiliary disorders in inflammatory bowel disease. *Surg. Gyn. Obstet.*, **160**, 187–93
14. Minuk, G.Y. (1988). Hepatobiliary complications of idiopathic inflammatory bowel disease. *Can. J. Gastroenterol.*, **2**, 109A–114A

15. Schrumpf, E., Fausa, O., Kolmannskog, F., Elgjo, K., Rittland, S. and Gjone, E. (1982). Sclerosing cholangitis in ulcerative colitis. A follow-up study. *Scand. Gastroenterol.*, **17**, 33–9
16. Seyrig, J.A., Jian, R., Modigliani, R., Golfain, D., Florent, C., Messing, B. and Bitoun, A. (1985). Idiopathic pancreatitis associated with inflammatory bowel disease. *Dig. Dis. Sci.*, **30**, 1121–6
17. Talbot, R.W., Heppell, J., Dozois, R.R. and Beart, R.W. (1986). Vascular complications of inflammatory bowel disease. *Mayo Clin. Proc.*, **61**, 140–5
18. Manomohan, V., Subbuswamy, S.G. and Willoughby, C.P. (1984). Crohn's disease and pericarditis. *Postgrad. Med. J.*, **60**, 682–4
19. Lowdell, C.P., Shousha, S., Path, M.R.C. and Parkins, R.A. (1986). The incidence of amyloidosis complicating inflammatory bowel disease. A prospective survey of 177 patients. *Dis. Col. Rect.*, **29**, 351–4
20. Hollander, D., Vadheim, C.M., Brettholz, E., Peterson, G.M., Delahunty, T.J. and Rotter, J. (1986). Increased intestinal permeability in Crohn's disease patients and their relatives: An etiological factor? *Ann. Intern. Med.*, **105**, 883–5
21. Glassman, M., Kaplan, M. and Spivak, W. (1986). Immune-complex glomerulonephritis in Crohn's disease. *J. Pediatr. Gastroenterol. Nutr.*, **5**, 966–9
22. Bush, A., Mitchison, H., Walt, R., Baron, J.H., Boylston, A.W. and Summerfield, J.A. (1987). Primary biliary cirrhosis and ulcerative colitis. *Gastroenterology*, **92**, 2009–13
23. Miller, B. (1980). Nebenwirkungen der Therapie mit Salazosulfapyridin. *Dtsch. Med. Wschr.*, **105**, 1596–7
24. Dew, M.J., van Berge Henegouwen, G.P., Huybregts, A.W.M. and Allan, R.N. (1980). Hepatotoxic effect of bile acids in inflammatory bowel disease. *Gastroenterology*, **78**, 1393–401
25. Holzbach, R.T., Marsh, M.E., Freedman, M.R., Fazio, V.W., Lavery, I.C. and Jagelman, D.A. (1980). Portal vein bile acids in patients with severe inflammatory bowel disease. *Gut*, **21**, 428–35
26. Chapman, R.W., Cottone, M., Selby, S.W., Shepherd, H.A., Sherlock, S. and Jewell, D.P. (1986). Serum autoantibodies, ulcerative colitis and primary sclerosing cholangitis. *Gut*, **27**, 86–91
27. Bjarnason, I., Zanelli, G., Smith, T., Prouse, P., Williams, P., Smethurst, P., Delacey, G., Gumpel, M.J. and Levi, A.J. (1987). Nonsteroidal antiinflammatory drug-induced intestinal inflammation in humans. *Gastroenterology*, **93**, 480–9
28. LaRusso, N.F., Wiesner, R.H., Ludwig, J. and MacCarty, R.L. (1984). Primary sclerosing cholangitis. *N. Engl. J. Med.*, **310**, 899–903
29. Patwardhan, R.V., Heilpern, J., Brewster, A.C. *et al.* (1983). Pleuropericarditis: An extraintestinal complication of inflammatory bowel disease. *Arch. Intern. Med.*, **143**, 94–6
30. Meyers, S., Greenspan, J., Greenstein, A.J., Cohen, B.A. and Janowitz, H.D. (1987). Pancreatitis coincident with Crohn's ileocolitis. Report of a case and review of the literature. *Dis. Col. Rect.*, **30**, 119–22
31. Compston, J.E., Judd, D., Crawley, E.O., Evans, W.D., Evans, C., Church, H.A., Reid, E.M. and Rhodes, J. (1987). Osteoporosis in patients with inflammatory bowel disease. *Gut*, **28**, 410–5
32. Driscoll, R.H., Meredith, S.C., Sitrin, M. and Rosenberg, I.H. (1982). Vitamin D deficiency and bone disease in patients with Crohn's disease. *Gastroenterology*, **83**, 1252–8
33. von Westarp, C., Thomson, A.B.R., Overton, T.R., Rogers, R.M., Hodges, P.E., Fornasier, V.L. and Crockford, P.M. (1987). Disorders of mineral and bone metabolism in patients with Crohn's disease. *Can. J. Gastroenterol.*, **1**, 11–17
34. Imes, S., Dinwoodie, A., Walker, K., Pinchbeck, B. and Thomson, A.B.R. (1976). Vitamin C status in 137 outpatients with Crohn's disease. *J. Clin. Gastroenterol.*, **8**, 443–6
35. Schölmerich, J., Becher, M-S., Hoppe-Seyler, P., Matern, S., Häussinger, D., Löhle, E., Köttgen, E. and Gerok, W. (1985). Zinc and vitamin A deficiency in patients with Crohn's disease is correlated with activity but not with localization or extent of disease. *Hepatogastroenterology*, **32**, 34–8

36. Ainley, C.C., Cason, J., Carlsson, L.K., Slavin, B.M. and Thomson, R.P.H. (1988). Zinc status in inflammatory bowel disease. *Clin. Sci.*, **75**, 277–83
37. Sjörgren, A., Florén, C-H. and Nilson, A. (1988). Evaluation of zinc status in subjects with Crohn's disease. *Am. J. Nutr.*, **7**, 57–60
38. Imes, S., Pinchbeck, B., Dinwoodie, A., Walker, K. and Thomson, A.B.R. (1987). Vitamin A status in 137 patients with Crohn's disease. *Digestion*, **37**, 166–70
39. Nishi, Y., Lifschitz, F., Bayne, M.A., Daum, F., Silverberg, M. and Aiges, H. (1980). Zinc status and its relation to growth retardation in children with chronic inflammatory bowel disease. *Am. J. Clin. Nutr.*, **33**, 2613–21
40. Balzer, K., Breuer, N., Hotz, J., Förster, S. and Goebell, H. (1984). Zur Genese von Hyposiderinämie and Anämie beim Morbus Crohn. *Dtsch. Med. Wschr.*, **109**, 1023–8
41. Lederer, P.C., Cidlinsky, K., Kobal, G. and Lux, G. (1985). Geschmacksstörungen bei M. Crohn-Patienten – Elektrogustometrie und chemische Geschmacksprüfung. *Z. Gastroenterol.*, **23**, 470
42. Kirschner, B.S., Klich, J.R., Kalman, S.S., De Favaro, M.V. and Rosenberg, I.H. (1981). Reversal of growth retardation in Crohn's disease with therapy emphasizing oral nutritional restitution. *Gastroenterology*, **80**, 10–15
43. Farthing, M.J.G. and Dawson, A.M. (1983). Impaired semen quality in Crohn's disease – drugs, ill health, or undernutrition? *Scand. J. Gastroenterol.*, **18**, 57–60
44. Solomons, N.W., Rosenberg, I.H., Sandstead, H.H. and Vo-Khactu, K.P. (1977). Zinc deficiency in Crohn's disease. *Digestion*, **16**, 87–95
45. Filipsson, S., Hultén, L. and Lindstedt, G. (1978). Malabsorption of fat and vitamin B_{12} before and after intestinal resection for Crohn's disease. *Scand. J. Gastroenterol.*, **13**, 529–36
46. Main, A.N.H., Mills, P.R., Russell, R.I., Bronte-Stewart, J., Nelson, L.M., McLeland, A. and Shenkin, A. (1983). Vitamin A deficiency in Crohn's disease. *Gut*, **24**, 1169–75
47. McClain, C., Su, L.C., Gilbert, H. and Cameron, D. (1983). Zinc-deficiency-induced retinal dysfunction in Crohn's disease. *Dig. Dis. Sci.*, **28**, 85–7
48. Andersson, H., Bosaeus, I., Fasth, S., Hellberg, R. and Hultén, L. (1987). Cholelithiasis and urolithiasis in Crohn's disease. *Scand. J. Gastroenterol.*, **22**, 253–6
49. Schölmerich, J., Braun, G., Volk, B.A., Spamer, C., Hoppe-Seyler, P. and Gerok, W. (1987). Detection of extraintestinal and intestinal abnormalities in inflammatory bowel disease by ultrasound. *Dig. Surg.*, **4**, 82–7
50. Dharmsathaphorn, K., Freeman, D.H., Binder, H.J. and Dobbins, J.W. (1982). Increased risk of nephrolithiasis in patients with steatorrhea. *Dig. Dis. Sci.*, **27**, 401–5
51. Matern, S. (1982). Chologene Diarrhoe und chologene Steatorrhoe. *Z. Allgmed.*, **58**, 601–7
52. Heumann, R., Sjödahl, R., Tobiasson, P. and Tagesson, C. (1982). Postprandial serum bile acids in resected and non-resected patients with Crohn's disease. *Scand. J. Gastroenterol.*, **17**, 137–40
53. Holmquist, L., Andersson, H., Rudic, N., Ahrén, C. and Fällström, P. (1986). Bile acid malabsorption in children and adolescents with chronic colitis. *Scand. J. Gastroenterol.*, **21**, 87–92
54. Rutgeerts, P., Ghoos, Y., Vantrappen, G. and Fevery, J. (1986). Biliary lipid composition in patients with nonoperated Crohn's disease. *Dig. Dis. Sci.*, **31**, 27–32
55. Tougaard, L., Giese, B., Højlund Pedersen, B. and Binder, V. (1986). Bile acid metabolism in patients with Crohn's disease in terminal ileum. *Scand J. Gastroenterol.*, **21**, 627–33
56. Müller, G., Schütte, W. and Möller, T. (1987). Pathogenese von Hyperoxalurien und Kalziumoxalatsteinen bei Darmerkrankungen. *Dtsch. Z. Verdau Stoffwechselkrankh*, **47**, 105–12
57. Greenstein, A.J. and Sacher, D.B. (1983). Cancer in inflammatory bowel disease. *Surv. Dig. Dis.*, **1**, 8–18
58. Greenstein, A.J., Gennuso, R., Sachar, D.B., Heimann, T., Smith, H., Janowitz, H.D. and Aufses, A.H. (1985). Extraintestinal cancers in inflammatory bowel disease. *Cancer*, **56**, 2914–21

59. Petras, R.E., Mir-Madjlessi, S.H. and Farmer, R.G. (1987). Crohn's disease and intestinal carcinoma. A report of 11 cases with emphasis on associated epithelial dysplasis. *Gastroenterology*, **93**, 1307–14
60. Mir-Madjlessi, S.H., Farmer, R.G. and Sivak, M.V. (1987). Bile duct carcinoma in patients with ulcerative colitis. Relationship to sclerosing cholangitis: Report of six cases and review of the literature. *Dig. Dis. Sci.*, **32**, 145–54

6
Current state of surgery in Crohn's disease

C. HERFARTH AND M. BETZLER

INTRODUCTION

The inflammatory bowel diseases – ulcerative colitis and Crohn's disease – differ not only with respect to pathohistological findings but also in the effects of surgical treatment. With ulcerative colitis there are ulcerative changes of the mucose membrane of the colorectal area which differ in regard to the state of the disease and the extent of the depth of inflammatory ulcerations. The entire bowel wall is involved in Crohn's disease by ulcerative fissures, fistulae, abscesses and stenoses, more usually located in the distal small bowel – but these may also appear in a multicentric manner throughout the gastrointestinal tract. Ulcerative colitis can be cured by resecting the affected bowel segment or the affected mucosa (rectum), respectively. With Crohn's disease the resection of affected bowel segments has a high recurrence rate due to the systemic pattern of the disease. The accepted indications for surgical treatment are disease-related complications or cases which cannot be controlled by consequent medical therapy. The indication for the necessary surgical procedure has to be decided for the individual patient as that moment determined to be suitable by a consensus between the internist (gastroenterologist) and the surgeon.

INDICATIONS FOR SURGERY

Surgical treatment in Crohn's disease is indicated when complications of the disease occur and there are systemic manifestations which cannot be influenced by the appropriate conservative therapeutic measures. Elective surgery in Crohn's disease is indicated after unsuccessful conservative therapy under the following findings:

Chronic recurrent obstruction
Bladder or urinary tract fistulae
Interenteric or enterocutaneous system of fistulae with possible abscesses
Reduced general state of health despite adequate conservative therapy.

The predictive value of the van Hees activity index[1] concerning the early diagnosis of septic complications in regard to the indication for surgery seems to be rather doubtful. Table 6.1 sets out the indications for surgery of the patients in our institution over the last 5 years; these figures correspond with those cited in the literature[2,3].

Table 6.1 Indications for operation in 272 patients with Crohn's disease[a]

Indications	*n*
Chronic obstruction	147
Fistulae	114
Urogenitary tract complications	17
Urgency	4
Other	41

[a] 10/1981–12/1986, Department of Surgery, University of Heidelberg

Absolute indications for surgery are perforation, peritonitis, non-treatable toxic megacolon, non-controllable bleeding and mechanical obstruction. However, experience has proved that a mechanical obstruction due to Crohn's disease is only very rarely an absolute indication for surgery – this is also true for bleeding in Crohn-affected bowel segments[4].

In the course of the chronic disease most Crohn's disease patients have to be operated on due to the complications that occur. The American MCCD Study[5] showed that between 80 and 90% of patients have to be operated on during a 20-year course of illness. The probability of surgical treatment varies in respect to the affected organ. The most frequent indication is involvement of the ileocaecal region; a less frequent indication is an exclusively affected large or small bowel segment.

OPERATIVE PROCEDURE

In the majority of cases the operative procedures in Crohn's disease have been restricted to small or large bowel resections (Table 6.2): by now most surgeons resect the affected bowel segment with a safe margin of 5 cm of macroscopic disease-free bowel. The risk of leaving a *macroscopically* affected bowel segment, which either results in a too short resection or in bypass operation without resection, lies in the persistency of the inflammatory state of the disease and the high recurrence rate. The results published by a number of authors[6,7] show more generous resection of 'healthy bowel' not to be necessary since even histologically Crohn-affected bowel with a macroscopically inconspicuous resection edge does not lead to worsening of the prognosis. Kyle[8] favoured the instant intraoperative pathological examination of the bowel segments which were intended for anastomosis, but this has not been accepted by the surgical community in recent years. A radical resection procedure in Crohn's disease has been put forward based on the idea that early extensive resection would cure Crohn's disease or at least drastically lower the recurrence rate[9], despite the risk of a short bowel syndrome. Meanwhile published results from the second German Crohn study[16] show that radical surgical procedures in comparison to restricted resection do not give any advantages with regard to the post-operative recurrence rate. These results correspond with Lee's findings[11]: there is nowadays no rationale for radical resection in Crohn's disease since it is not curable by resection. This appraisal also accords with the patho-morphological observation that the total intestinum can be affected in Crohn's disease with varying intensity of the inflammatory process[12].

Table 6.2 Operative procedures in patients with Crohn's disease[a]

Operations	*n*
Colon resection (including ileocaecal resection)	144
Small bowel resection	142
Fistula-Op without intestinal resection	54
Stricture-plasty	26[b]
Omentum-plasty	22
Other	43

[a] 10/1981–12/1986, Department of Surgery, University of Heidelberg
[b] In eight patients

It is well known that prospective randomized controlled studies are the best way of judging (by therapeutic measurements) the optimal extent of resection in Crohn's disease. However, it must be stated that up to now no such study has been reported in the literature. Instead most reports on recurrence rate are retrospective analyses concerning more or less extensive resection procedures with only small case numbers and a relatively short follow-up time. A further problem is how to define a Crohn's disease relapse: microscopically, macroscopically, by endoscopy, by X-ray, or clinically.

Heumann[13] was able to prove in his study that the recurrence rate is at present increasingly independent of the microscopic evidence of Crohn's disease in the resection edges. In his analysis, the relapse rate was 36% for patients with Crohn-free resection edges in comparison to 38% of patients with microscopically evident Crohn's disease in the resection edges. Other authors[14,15] confirm these results though others such as Wolff[9], Nygaard[16] and Karesen[17] report contrary results.

Summing up these differing results and observations we can conclude that chronic disease persists even after resection and independently of its extent. It can also be concluded that microscopic changes due to Crohn's disease are already detectable at the time of resection in those parts of the gastrointestinal tract which were macroscopically disease-free. Accordingly, Lee[11] postulated that the recurrence rate is dependent on the natural history of the disease rather than on the surgical procedure. This evaluation supports the concept of so-called 'minimal surgery'[18] which includes short segment resection and procedures such as stricture-plasty. This last mentioned method was first described by Lee[18] and confirmed by Alexander-Williams[19] and Hawker[20] with reference to larger series of patients. Nevertheless, the stricture-plasty is restricted to only a minority of Crohn's disease patients since only circumscribed stenoses are suitable for this method. However, the results with limited and non-resecting operative techniques prove that the predominant aim of surgical measures in Crohn's disease is to abolish the typical complications.

According to our experience the following principles for surgical treatment of Crohn's disease have proved successful:

(1) restrictive resection;

(2) performance of an end-to-end anastomosis with a one-layer suture technique;

(3) use of drainage only in very special cases (with the idea that foreign body reaction favours relapse).

These principles are accepted if only the small bowel or the ileocaecal region are affected. But there are diverging opinions on the treatment if the colon is diffusely affected: whether to perform a proctocolectomy or a colectomy with ileorectal anastomosis. The criteria for sphincter-preserving colectomy with ileorectal anastomoses are patients with sphincter continence without complicating anal fistulae and with little or no Crohn's disease changes in the rectum. According to these criteria only about one half of the mostly young patients with Crohn's disease colitis are eligible for the sphincter-preserving procedure, while in the rest of the patients a proctocolectomy or a colectomy with a terminal ileostomy and blindly closed rectal stump have to be performed[21]. In larger studies, on ileorectal anastomoses with a follow-up time of 10 years, a cumulative relapse rate between 40 and 64% and a cumulative reoperation rate between 40 and 50% were found[21,22]. These figures are acceptable, especially if they are compared to data for ileocaecal resection at those institutions with a relapse and reoperation rate of 40 and 30%, respectively.

In our own group of Crohn's disease patients, with a median follow-up time of 6 years, the cumulative relapse rate was 39% and the reoperation rate 30%. The coincidence of anal lesions with large and small bowel affected by Crohn's disease lies between 10 and 30% for Crohn-affected small bowel and between 50 and 80% for Crohn-affected large bowel[23,24].

Crohn's disease isolated to the terminal ileum occurs less frequently in the literature today than it did 30–40 years ago[12]; but even less frequent is isolated Crohn's disease involvement of the colon. Isolated Crohn's disease of the colon is characterized by frequent diarrhoea and less frequently by relapsing obstructive symptoms which are more typical for Crohn's diseaes in the small bowel. Limited resection is indicated if only a segment of the colon is affected. Mekhjian[5] was able to show that the prognosis of the disease is worse if both small and large bowel are affected.

Lock[25] could demonstrate in a controlled study that the relapse rate within a 10-year follow-up after resection depends on the primary location in the small bowel, the ileocaecal region, or the colon, and lies between 20 and 40%. In the same series of patients reoperation was necessary for every third patient. In spite of the high relapse incidence one should always keep in mind that the remission time after surgical procedures is considerably longer than after conservative treatment – as was shown by Hulten[26]. Of all Hulten's patients 70% spent years in full clinical remission after surgical procedures in comparison to less than 20% after conservative treatment.

CROHN'S DISEASE FISTULAE

It must be regarded as a basic principle in the treatment of Crohn's disease fistulae that the procedure must be differentiated, individualized and as conservative as possible. In Table 6.3 the distribution of the different types of enteric fistulae are shown for our own group of 95 patients. Perianal fistulae in Crohn's disease show a high rate of asymptomatic fistulae and spontaneous healing, but also a considerable recurrence rate[27,28]. Occasionally fistulae prove to heal at least partially after proximal resection of the intestine[24]. As for perianal Crohn's disease fistulae it can be stated that their incidence amounts to about 25% when the small bowel is affected whereas it rises to about 100% when the rectum is affected[24,29]. Perianal fistulae prove to be the sole clinical manifestation of Crohn's diseaes in only 5%; nevertheless in 9–24% of patients they are the first symptom of Crohn's disease[30]. For rectovaginal fistula, surgery is only indicated if subjective symptoms are present. In cases of anal or rectal stenosis due to Crohn's disease good results could be obtained by endoscopic laser treatment[31].

Table 6.3 Distribution of operated enteric fistulae in 95 patients with Crohn's disease[a]

Enteric fistula	*%*
Interenteric	45
Enterocutaneous	19
Perianal	28
Recto-vaginal	4
Entero-vesical	4
Combined	20

[a] 10/1981–12/1985, Department of Surgery, University of Heidelberg

SUMMARY

As the majority of patients with Crohn's disease have to be operated on during the course of their disease, the indication for surgery should be the result of an interdisciplinary agreement between the internist and the surgeon, taking into consideration the circumstances of the individual patient's long-term course of illness. In recent years a growing tendency for early operation can be noted because conservative treatment, which lasts either too long or fails, can possibly lead to additional complications or aggravation of symptoms, respectively.

The tendency to intervene surgically at an early stage seems to be neither more nor less justified by under 1% low mortality rates[3]. Realizing that Crohn's disease cannot be cured surgically, it must be concluded that resecting treatment must be very restrictive, i.e. only for such segments of the intestine as are macroscopically affected. The patients' quality of life can best be improved by such a therapeutical regimen. In view of the high recurrence rate it has become the rule to operate more restrictively but also more frequently.

REFERENCES

1. Van Hees, P.A.M., van Elteren, P.H., van Lier, H.J.J. and Tongeren, J.H.M. (1980). An index of inflammatory activity in patients with Crohn's diseaes. *Gut*, **21**, 279–86
2. Fazio, V.W. and Turnbull, R.B. (1980). Ulcerative colitis and Crohn's disease of the colon: a review of surgical options. *Med. Clin. North Am.*, **64**, 1135–59
3. Herfarth, Ch. and Betzler, M. (1985). Indikation und chirurgische Verfahrenswahl bei Colitis ulcerosa und Morbus Crohn. In: Ewe, K. and Fahrländer, H. (eds.) *Therapie chronisch entzündlicher Darmerkrankungen*. (Stuttgart/New York: Schattauer), pp. 177–189
4. Hersfarth, Ch. (1978). Morbus Crohn – Indikation zur Operation. *Leber Magen. Darm.*, **8**, 212–7
5. Mekhjian, H.S., Switz, D.M., Watts, H.D., Deren, J., Katon, R.M. and Beman, F.M. (1979). The national co-operative Crohn's disease study. *Gastroenterology*, **77**, 907–13
6. Herfarth, Ch. (1983). Chronisch-entzündliche Darmerkrankungen – Indikation zur Operation. *Z. Gastroenterol.*, **21**, 27–34
7. Pennington, L., Hamilton, S.R., Bayless, T.M. and Cameron, J.L. (1980). Surgical management of Crohn's disease. *Ann. Surg.*, **192**, 311–8
8. Kyle, J.. (1972). Surgical treatment of Crohn's disease of the small intestine. *Br. J. Surg.*, **59**, 821–3
9. Wolff, B.G., Beart, R.W., Frydenberg, H.B. *et al.* (1983). The importance of disease-free margins in resection for Crohn's disease. *Dis. Colon Rectum*, **26**, 239–43
10. Herfarth, Ch. and Ewe, K. (1989). Chirurgisch-internistische Therapiestudie über die postoperative Rezidivprophylaxe des Morbus Crohn. (In press)
11. Lee, E.C.G. (1984). Aim of surgical treatment of Crohn's disease. *Gut*, **25**, 217–22
12. Dyer, N.H. (1970). Reply to: How regional is enteritis? *Gastroenterology*, **58**, 415
13. Heuman, R., Boeryd, B., Bolin, T. and Sjödahl, R. (1983). The influence of disease at the margin of resection on the outcome of Crohn's disease. *Br. J. Surg.*, **70**, 519–21
14. Hamilton, S.R., Bussey, H.J.R. and Boitnott, J.K. (1981). Active inflammation and granulomas in grossly uninvolved colonic mucosa of Crohn's disease resection specimens studied with an face histologic technique. *Gastroenterology*, **80**, 1167 (Abstract)
15. Papaiannaou, N., Piris, J. and Lee, E.C.G. (1979). The relationship between histologic inflammation in the cut ends after resection of Crohn's disease and recurrence. *Gut*, **20**, A916
16. Nygaard, K. and Fausa, O. (1977). Crohn's disease. *Scand. J. Gastroenterol.*, **12**, 577–84
17. Karesen, R., Serch-Hanssen, A., Thoresen, B.O. and Hertzberg, J. (1981). Crohn's disease: Long-term results of surgical treatment. *Scand. J. Gastroenterol.*, **16**, 57–64
18. Lee, E.C.G. and Papaioannou, N. (1982). Minimal surgery for chronic obstruction in patients with extensive or universal Crohn's disease. *Ann. R. Coll. Surg. Engl.*, **64**, 229–33
19. Alexander-Williams, J. and Fornaro, M. (1982). Stricture-plasty beim Morbus Crohn. *Chirurgie*, **53**, 799–801
20. Hawker, P.C., Allan, R.N., Dykes, P.W. and Alexander-Williams, J. (1983). Strictureplasty. A useful, effective surgical treatment in Crohn's disease. *Gut*, **24**, A490
21. Alexander-Williams, J. and Buchmann, P. (1980). Criteria of assessment for suitability and results of ileorectal anastomosis. *Clin. Gastroenterol.*, **9**, 409–17
22. Ambrose, N.S., Keighley, M.R.B., Alexander-Williams, J. and Allan, R.N. (1984). Clinical impact of colectomy and ileorectal anastomosis in the management of Crohn's disease. *Gut*, **25**, 223–7
23. Buchmann, P., Wetermann, I., Keighley, M.R.B., Pena, S.A., Allan, R.N. and Alexander-Williams, J. (1981). The prognosis of ileorectal anastomosis in Crohn's disease. *Br. J. Surg.*, **68**, 7–10
24. Herfarth, Ch. and Bindewald, H. (1986). Perianale Erkrankung beim Morbus Crohn. *Chirurgie*, **57**, 304–8
25. Lock, M.R., Farmer, R.G., Fazio, V.W., Jagelmann, D.G., Lavery, I.C. and Weakley, F.L. (1981). Recurrence and reoperation for Crohn's disease. *N. Engl. J. Med.*, **304**, 1568–8
26. Hulten, L. (1979). Frühoperation beim Morbus Crohn, ja oder nein? *Internist*, **20**, 171–5

27. Hellers, G., Bergstrand, O. Ewerth, S. and Holmström, B. (1980). Occurrence and outcome after primary treatment of anal fistulae in Crohn's disease. *Gut*, **21**, 525
28. Marks, C.G., Ritchie, J.E. and Lockhart-Mummery, H.E. (1981). Anal fistulae in Crohn's disease. *Br. J. Surg.*, **68**, 525
29. Gross, E. and Eigler, F.W. (1983). Die Indikation zur lokalchirurgischen Therapie analer Manifestationen des Morbus Crohn. *Langenbecks Arch. Chir.*, **359**, 75
30. Alexander-Williams, J. and Buchmann, P. (1980). Perianal Crohn's disease. *World J. Surg.*, **4**, 203–8
31. Friedl, P. and Betzler, M. (1986). Erste Erfahrungen mit dem Einsatz des Neodym-YAG Lasers bei benignen Rektumstenosen. *Colo-proctology*, **No. 6**, 347

Index

MIX
Papier aus verantwortungsvollen Quellen
Paper from responsible sources
FSC® C105338

If you have any concerns about our products,
you can contact us on
ProductSafety@springernature.com

In case Publisher is established outside the EU,
the EU authorized representative is:
Springer Nature Customer Service Center GmbH
Europaplatz 3, 69115 Heidelberg, Germany

Printed by Libri Plureos GmbH
in Hamburg, Germany